A Beautiful You.
The 30~Day Detox Program

Your 30~Day Guide To A Spectacular You!

Dianna P. Riley

FOR YOUR FREE HEALTH HISTORY,

GO TO:

http://www.holisticlifestylechanges.com/

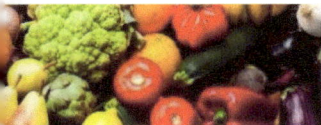

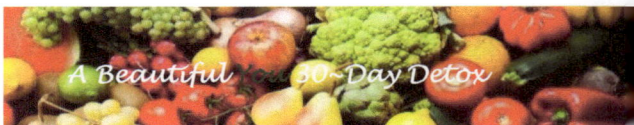

The content herein.

DISCLAIMER AND/OR LEGAN NOTICES:

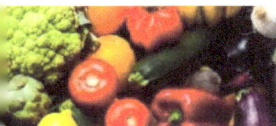

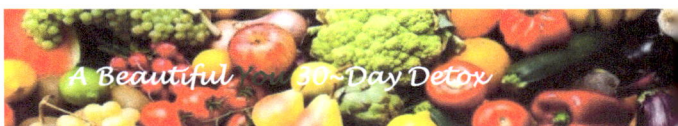

Table of Contents

The content herein. 1

THE REASON I WROTE THIS BOOK 16

Chapter 1 – Detoxing: Why? 17

Chapter 2 – What A Detox Does For You! 19

    Detox At anytime... 19

Chapter 3 – Putting Your Detox Fears to Rest 21

    FAQ's – Easing Your Detox Fears 21

Chapter 4 – Probiotics and Cultured Foods............. 24

    The What & How of Probiotics 24

    As Well As Cultured Foods 25

Chapter 5 – Get a Better Understanding of the Elimination Diet 27

    Pre-Tox Instructions 27

    Detox Instructions 28

    Detox Transition Instructions 28

    Your Food Journal – Writing It All Down 29

Chapter 6 – What Level Are You? 31

Chapter 7 – Making Preparations & Planning For Your Detox... 34

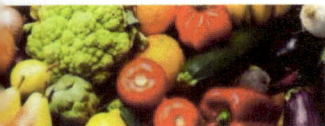

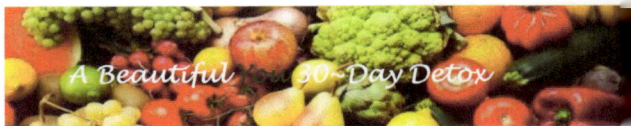

How to Prep 34

The Pre-Tox 34

Elimination List 35

Successful Detox Tips 35

The Emotional Facets of Detoxing and Weight Loss
.... 36

Chapter 8 - The Daily To-Do List for Detoxing 38

Have Fun Planning Your Meals 39

Juicing While Detoxing 39

Drinking to Flush Out the Toxins 39

Chapter 9 – Your Detox Program 41

Day One 41

Day Two 41

Day Three 42

Day Four 42

Day Five 42

Day Six 43

Day Seven 43

Day Eight 43

Day Nine 43

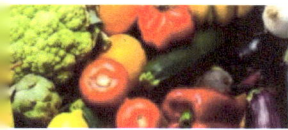

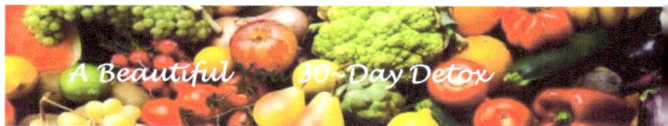

Day Ten 44

Day Eleven 44

Day Twelve 44

Day Thirteen 44

Day Fourteen 45

Day Fifteen 45

Day Sixteen 45

Day Seventeen 45

Day Eighteen 46

Day Nineteen 46

Day Twenty 46

Day Twenty-One 46

Day Twenty-Two 47

Day Twenty-Three 47

Day Twenty-Four 47

Day Twenty-Five 47

Day Twenty-Six 48

Chapter 10 – Your Transition 49

Your Food Diary 49

Chapter 11 – Your Transition Diet 51

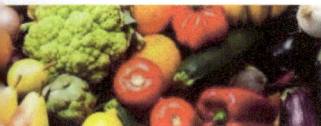

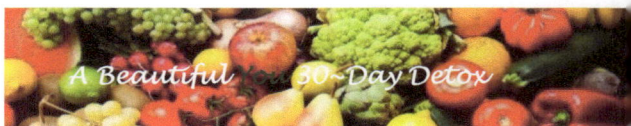

Day 1 51

Day 2 51

Day 3 51

Day 4 52

YOU'VE JUST FINISHED YOUR TRANSITION DIET AND DETOX! 52

Chapter 12 – Detox I Feel Greats! 54

Hot Towel Scrubs 54

Nourishments for Your Skin 55

Physical Activity 55

Hydration 55

Do Something Rewarding For Yourself Every Day 55

Rewrite Your Inner Narrative 56

A Great Epsom Salt Bath 56

Castor Oil Packets 56

Chapter 13 – Your Detox Meal Recipes 58

Fantabulous Smoothies! 58

Thin Mint Fat Busting Smoothie 58

Black & Strawberry Dreamcicle Smoothie 58

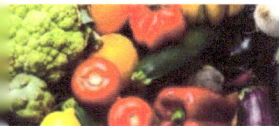

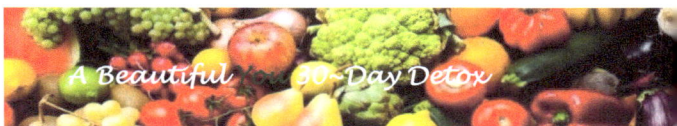

Creaminess with a lil' Kick 58

Chocolate Covered Cherries 58

Greased Lightning Smoothie 59

Sassy RAW Smoothie 59

Thunderbolt with a Dash of Sunshine 59

Sleek & Sassy Smoothie 59

Summer of Love Smoothie 59

Pear of Lovers Green Smoothie 60

Pineapple Orange Delight Smoothie 60

Banana – Mango Tropics Smoothie 60

Orange – Cantaloupe Hit the Tropics Smoothie .. 60

Banilla – Orange Smoothie 60

Carrot – Apricot Delight Smoothie 60

Fruity Zucchini Smoothie 61

Banananza Smoothie 61

Smoothie with a Kick 61

Apple Delight 61

Happy Cucumber "N" Melon Smoothie 61

Cantaloupe Delight Smoothie 61

Simply Nourishing Smoothie 62

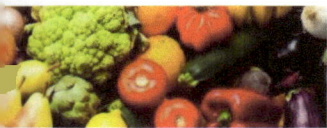

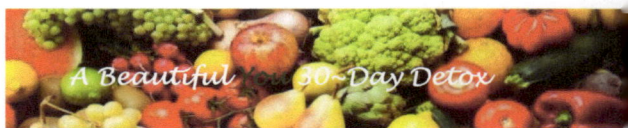

Great Day-In-The-Morning Smoothie 62

Peachy – Keen Smoothie 62

Papapple Smoothie 62

Banana – Strawberry Smoothie 62

Mango Tango Smoothie 62

Orange Madness Smoothie 63

Vanilla – Pineapple Sunrise Smoothie 63

Juicing 64

Hydration Station 64

Luscious Skin Green Goodness 64

Let's Go Wild 64

Not your Momma's Green Juice 64

Goodness Gracious Green Juice 65

Mean Green Mojito 65

The Anti-Wrinkle Green Juice 65

Cucumber – Grapefruit Juice 65

Flowing Digestion Juice 65

Oh My Healthy Liver 66

DIPS 67

Tahini Dip 67

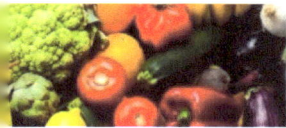

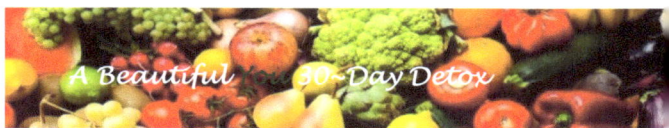

Raw Bean Free Hummus.. 67

Mexicali Dip... 67

Detoxing Pesto 67

Peach Salsa 68

Sweet Potato – Sage Dip 68

RAW MEALS.. 69

Detox Your Body Lettuce Wraps 69

Tomato – Fennel Salad 69

Beach Body Slaw 69

Mistress of the Citrus Salad 69

Orange ~ Arugula Salad... 70

Sweet & Sexy Detox Salad...................................... 70

Dijon Corn Salad.. 70

Delicious Asian Salad.. 70

Warm Spinach Salad 71

Minty Watermelon Salad 71

Lavish Berry Salad with Ginger Pineapple Dressing
.... 71

Fruity Zucchini Salad 72

Mediterranean Kale Salad 72

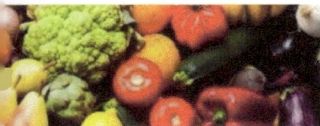

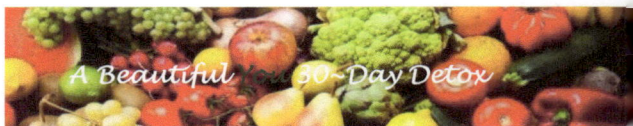

Cress Salad with Golden Beets 72

Raw Pasta with Marinara 72

Jicama Salad with Smashing Curry Sauce 73

Smashing Curry Sauce 73

Luscious Summer Salad 73

BRITTLE: 73

THE SALAD 74

Peachy Kale Salad with Miso Vinaigrette 74

VINAIGRETTE: 74

Berry ~ Mango Salad 74

BLUEBERRY VINAIGRETTE: 74

Luscious Melon Salad with Mint 74

Heirloom Tomatoes with a Mexi ~ Cali Salad 75

MEXI ~ CALI DRESSING: 75

Dressed Up Zucchini with Veggies 75

MARINADE: 75

MUSHROOMS: 75

Maple Dancing on the Tongue Slaw 76

SLAW: 76

MAPLE DRESSING: 76

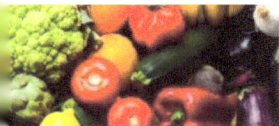

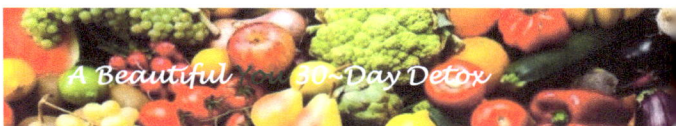

Carrot Curry Salad.. 76

CURRY DRESSING: 76

Marinated Cucumbers... 76

MARINADE:.. 77

The Radish Has it Salad with Curry Vinaigrette. 77

SALAD:... 77

DRESSING:.. 77

COOKED MEALS.. 78

Healthy Bowl with Orange Zest............................. 78

Curried Butternut Squash with Broccoli.............. 78

Coconut Brussels Sprouts with Golden Beets 78

Spicy Tex ~ Mex Wrap 78

Confetti Rice 79

RAW SOUPS 80

Yummy Raw Tomato Bisque 80

Love Your Skin Soup.. 80

Not Yo Momma's Chicken Soup (Vegan)............. 80

Cream of Spinach Soup 81

Creamy Carrot Soup 81

Spicy Bok Choy ~ Coconut Soup 81

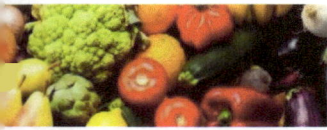

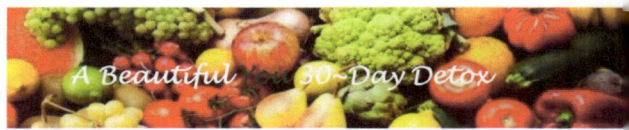

HOT CHILI GARLIC SAUCE 82

Raw Tomato Basil Soup 82

Cream of Asparagus Soup........................... 82

Vietnamese Pho Soup 82

Butternut Squash Soup 83

Tomato Gazpacho Soup 83

Bonus Soup! Raw Dilly Chilled Mango Green Soup
.... 84

WARM SOUPS 84

Hot Butternut Squash Soup 84

**Sea Vegetable Soup with Miso and Shitake
Mushrooms** 84

Food for the Soul Soup 85

Hindi Sweet Potato Soup 85

Cream of Cauliflower Soup......................... 86

Savory Red Lentil Soup.............................. 86

Ginger ~ Kale Soup with Miso.................... 86

DRESSINGS 88

Tahini Dressing 88

Honey Lemon Dressing............................... 88

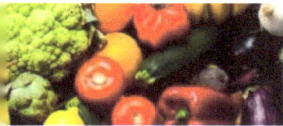

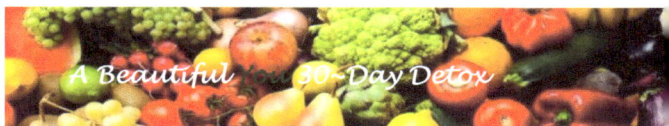

Oil and Vinegar with a Kick 88

Pineapple ~ Ginger Dressing................................. 88

Simple Miso Dressing 88

SNACKS 90

Trail Mix 90

Stuffed Fig or Date... 90

Kale Chips.. 90

Sweet Potato Delight 90

That Chocolate Thing You Do 90

Fancy Avocado 91

Delectable Sweet Potato.. 91

The Beverage Center 91

Banana Ecstasy... 91

Purse Treat 91

Collard Wraps with Turmeric Spread.................. 91

Sun ~ Dried Tomatoes Dressed in Green 91

Zucchini Steamboats.. 92

Scrumptious Poppers... 92

Lemony Cups.. 92

Dilly Stuffed Tomatoes 93

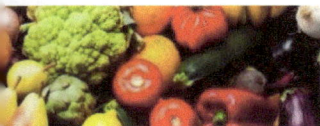

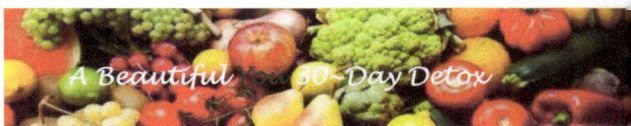

Tea Sandwiches in the Raw.................................... 93

Ants on a Log... 93

Banana ~ Tahini Celery Delight 94

TRANSITION RECIPES 95

SuperFood Quinoa Breakfast Bowl....................... 95

Organic Breakfast Bowl 95

Italian Hummus 95

Moroccan Quinoa Salad 95

SuperFood Goji Balls... 96

Butternut Squash Bowl... 96

Asparagus ~ Quinoa Risotto 97

Moroccan Spiced Bowl 97

DESSERTS 98

Raw Pudding 98

Creamsicle 98

Spice of Life Oatmeal Drink 98

Fruity Chia Dessert.. 98

Blackberry Sorbet.. 99

Mixed Berry Sorbet 99

Simply Yum Mix – Up... 99

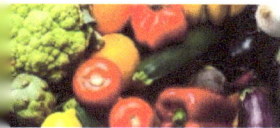

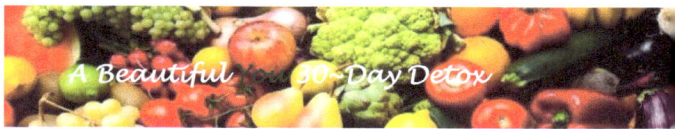

Your Chocolate Moment 99

BONUS DESSERTS – POST TRANSITION GUILTLESS SWEETS 99

Chocolate Moonlight Guiltless Balls 99

Sleepy Time Milkshake.. 100

Yummy Quinoa 'N' Milk 100

Chapter 14 – Articles You'll Need Along the Way 101

JOURNALING – WRITE YOURSELF THIN TO THE BODY YOU DESIRE! 101

PRE – TOX 101

DETOX 102

TRANSITION DAYS 102

What is a Big Picture Vision Board?................... 103

YOUR DAILY MOTIVATION FOR DETOX & WEIGHT LOSS 104

21 Daily Assertions To Love Yourself Into The Body You Long For! 104

LOW GLYCEMIC FOODS 106

SHOPPING LIST.. 109

YOUR DAILY FOOD DIARY 111

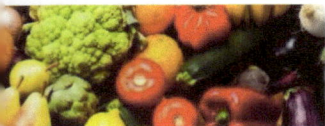

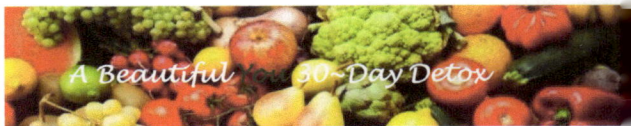

EATING OUT MADE EASY 116

DRINK YOURSELF THIN WITH PROBIOTICS
.... 119

STAGING THE KITCHEN 121

ABOUT THE AUTHOR 124

KUDOS AND THANK YOUS 127

DEDICATION 127

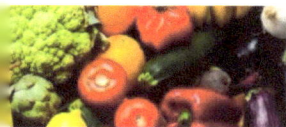

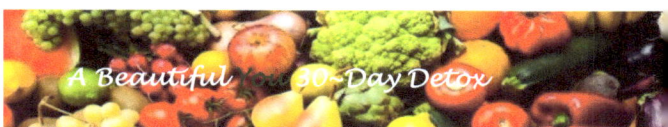

THE REASON I WROTE THIS BOOK

Writing this book was very personal for me! I've suffered with illnesses, struggled with my weight, and was ignorant as to how to really lose weight! I looked to every easy fix and quick pill, only to gain the weight back…rapidly! I see so many people making that same mistake all too often! This book as well as the program is for them.

I've tried so many fad diets only to have the weight come back, doubled in some instances. I was at a total loss and didn't know what to do or how to handle the unwanted weight. I siked or fooled myself into thinking that it was glandular or, everyone in my family on my dad's side is fat or big, so for a while, I even stopped trying to do anything about my weight.

One day, I was passing by a building with reflective windows and saw what everyone else saw and I was mortified! How could I let myself go that far? I had neighborhood kids call Ms. Fatty, or worse. I even tried buying "Slimming" clothing. Well, that didn't work!

It wasn't till I tried amphetamines, thinking that I was doing the smart thing. Well at the time I was taking them, I did lose the weight that I wanted only to gain it back after I stopped taking them.

My taking the amphetamines had a long lasting, negative effect on my health though. Right now, I suffer from Pulmonary Arterial Hypertension, (PAH) a very dangerous condition that causes narrowing of the arteries leading to the right lung. I'm now limited on the type of exercises that I can do, therefore, the weight loss was slow.

I found out about detoxing as well as eating raw! Now I'm not going to tell you the only way to become healthy is to eat totally raw, and my intentions are not to scare you away. But it wasn't until I embarked on this 30~Day Detox journey that I started feeling better. As a Certified Holistic Health Coach, I was able to put into practice what I'd learned from the Institute of Integrative Nutrition and have lost a tremendous amount of weight.

My goal is to get people like yourself healthier and happier, one person at a time while having fun detoxing your body. Please enjoy reading this book and hopefully, doing this delicious detox!

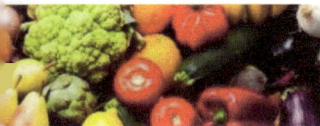

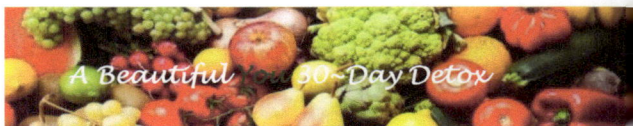

Chapter 1 – Detoxing: Why?

Welcome to your 'A Spectacular You: 30~Day Detox Program! You'll be so thrilled at the changes in your body and how you feel once you detox on this program. This 30~Day Detox will properly cleanse your body and when you properly cleanse your body, your body will release all of the toxins that rob you of your energy, you'll have a permanent glow about yourself and most importantly, you'll lose those some of those unwanted pounds with ease! Speaking from experience, I know how it feels to want to look and feel your best, I want that for you too. You'll find that you'll be waking up feeling fantabulous. So, everyday I'd love it if you were feeling and looking your best, enjoy yourself and have a wonderful glow – inside out!

When your body holds on to toxins, it becomes very toxic. A toxic body cannot digest food properly. In order to lose weight, proper digestion is key. It's the key to also maintaining an ideal weight too. Have you ever tried every diet on the market, like so many of us has, and nothing worked or it was a temporary fix? Well, if so, that is a great sign that it is time to do a detox. This 30~Day Detox will not only flush out the toxic waste effectively, it will allow you to ditch fad diets forever. Are you ready because this is just the beginning!

Your body truly does need as well as crave a perfect balance, so get ready because YOU are about to embark on a journey through which you will gain a better understanding of the connection between foods you eat, the beauty you possess, and the way you feel in your body when it is balanced. The strong guiding principles for this 30~Day Detox are:

- To improve your digestion
- Get rid of or eliminate the foods that may be causing you unwanted bloat
- Gradually reintroduce the right foods to get you and keep you feeling 10 years younger

Are you excited yet?! Well, get ready to be! I promise that you are going to have loads of fun. Whether you've done a cleanse in the past or you're a newbie, the 30~Day Detox Program is going to be a great start for you, no matter your level! Later in this guide, you'll find that there are three different Levels for the 30~Day Detox, depending on your health practices and the diet that you're on now. I feel confident that you'll find that you're on one of them. Find the cleansing level where you are for the 30~Day Detox and embrace the program. And don't worry if you're a newbie. Cleansing just means that you are going

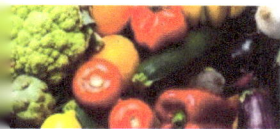

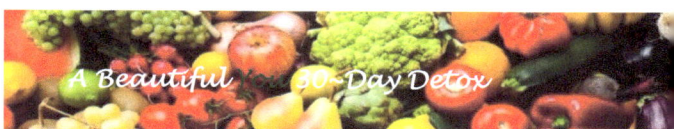

to clean out the gook and junk hanging out in your body, in a natural and healthy way. It's also going to be in an easy approach to get your body running like a fine tuned engine. And don't worry, no one will be there to judge you because there's no right or wrong here. Start at the level that suits you. You can do this! Always keep that in mind!

So, let's start this 30~Day Detox Program with your goals in mind. Write them down at this very moment on a piece of paper. You are cleansing for three reasons: More beauty (the inside beauty leads outside), boundless energy, and realizing the healthy body you are wanting and deserving. It's summertime after all, summer time means getting sexy for those bathing suits or swimming trunks, time at the beach, the pool or park – time for you to romp around, healthy and happy. This 30~Day Detox Program is going to get you where you want to be with a simple day-by-day, step-by-step plan so you don't have to stress out about how to go about how or what to eat. So just be calm, comfortable and prepared for your delicious journey ahead.

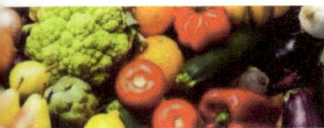

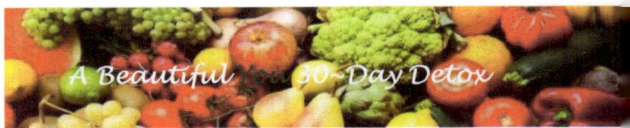

Chapter 2 – What A Detox Does For You!

Detox At anytime

When you think of summer, you think fresh, active and fun. It's the time to play, leg go and free up your mind and body. This time to get the body that you desire and deserve! Go for it! Take some time to reflect on the enjoyment of summertime. The trees have bloomed, the seasonal fruits are ripe, juicy and scrumptious, plus the entire season is packed with wholesome, fun activities. This is the one season that encourages your body to lighten up and feel free. Are you prepared to laugh, do cartwheels like you were a kid again?

Have you noticed that in the summer, your appetite lightens up tremendously and you crave cooler foods like melons fresh fruits and raw salads? Well you can do just that and make it super fun and enjoyable. What you are going to experience is the foods that are in season, foods that promote natural detoxification, and foods that promote a healthy weight loss. Please keep in mind that your 30~Day Detox Program is not just about the next 30 days. My goal is to educate you so that the information and habits that you take away from this program will continue to be a positive and effective tool for the rest of your life!

Did you know that in Chinese medicine, summertime focuses on the element of fire? That's because fire encourages energy, vitality and growth. At this time, we will nourish and detox your heart and the small intestines. Your heart pumps 3,000 gallons of blood daily to the lungs, which is then absorbed as oxygen. Don't you think that now is the time to show your heart some love. Your heart also helps you on an emotional level to dream, and make those dreams a reality. Now is a great time to embrace your most powerful self and dream big! One way to start is by writing down those dreams in your daily journal because this will keep you focused with a clear view on what you have in store for yourself. Always keep in mind that your heart controls your whole body. It's the Warrior, the Empress, the King or Queen of your castle, and it deserves to be nourished and supported. Not only are you about to support your body better on a physical level, but also on an emotional one also.

The small intestine is vital in the detoxification process as 70% of your immune system in housed in it. The small intestine has an enormous job because it digests and absorbs all of your food. Then it sends the nutrients into the bloodstream, where they are carried to the liver and then transformed into energy. If your digestion is sluggish or if the lining of your

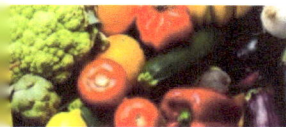

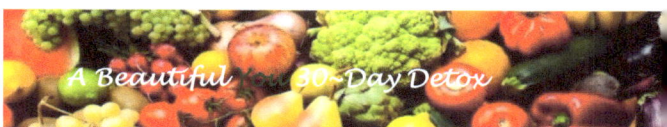

gut is damaged, that means that you are not absorbing your nutrients, which leads to a lack of energy that your body needs and deserves.

Your body has the ability to heal itself and run like a fine tuned racecar! You're a top notch machine. A better knowledge of the basic systems that are running you, the machine, is the most successful means to ditch the weight plus lose that nasty toxicity attached to your intestines. My goal is to enable you to be the expert on what works for your particular body and what it really needs to function at a superior level!

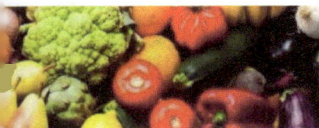

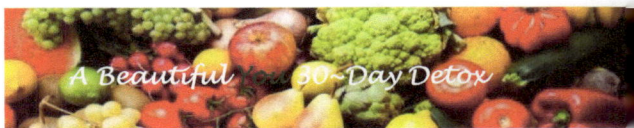

Chapter 3 – Putting Your Detox Fears to Rest

FAQ's – Easing Your Detox Fears

1. **Since the meals are already pre-planned for a specific day, can I choose another recipe or meal plan for another day?**

   Yes, just refer to the recipe section of this book and choose the recipe to exchange meals with. This is only a guide and you don't have to stick to specific days. If you have food intolerances to specific foods or you just don't like a specific recipe, you are free to do a swap out. Just don't choose anything from the transitional meals and stay within that detox phase of the program.

2. **If I have a headache/feel nauseated/am constipated, am I doing something wrong?**

   No, you aren't doing anything wrong. Those symptoms along with tiredness and emotional mood swings are all common effects of the detox process. This is the gunk and garbage coming out of your body. It's imperative that you drink enough water and add lemon and lime to improve liver function. Just like having sore muscles after a vigorous workout, these symptoms may be part of the process. Please make sure that, even during the Pre-Detox, that you are practicing your Detox Feel-Goods because even the Pre-Tox phase can produce a lot of detoxing, depending what level you're at. Make sure to listen to your body, this is very important! If your detoxification process is going too fast, slow it down a little. If you choose to detox with a friend or two, go just doing this detox at home alone, just stop for one day and let your body play catch-up. There are no right or wrong when it comes to listening and honoring your precious body.

3. **If I'm nursing, can I still follow the 30~Day Detox Program?**

   Sure, but make sure that you, before you do any kind of detox program, always check with your doctor and let him know what you're doing as it not only affects you, but also your baby. Add an additional 4 ounces of high quality protein (organic, free range animal or plant based) at breakfast, lunch and dinner. I also suggest you having an extra snack every day. (Refer to the Snack Section of this book).

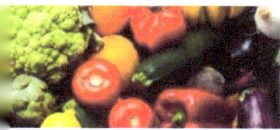

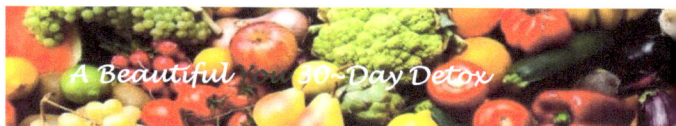

4. **If I attend a party, what do I eat?**

    This Detox Program is all about simple, clean eating. If going to a party or gathering, try and opt for an easy choice like a healthy salad with lemon and oil. Or you may have your fill before leaving home, so all you need to do, is piddle and mix. But if you prefer eating whilst at the party, try adding 3 to 4 ounces of clean, lean protein to your meal like shrimp, fish, chicken or a plant based protein as well as ½ of an avocado. Remember to just do your best while you're at a party or have to eat out at a restaurant to eat clean. This program is NOT about worrying your mind or body over what you should or shouldn't have. My main goal with this Detox Program is to remove this stress!

5. **Can I still do my exercises and workouts?**

    Yes! By all means if you have the energy you can still workout. Some folks detox and have a surmountable amount of energy. This is what I call a 'Detox High'. For others, a detox doesn't give them the endless amount of energy, leaving them feeling less energized. Remember that a detox can cause some dehydration, so make sure that you're drinking enough water. Try adding 1/8 tsp of high quality sea salt and stevia to your water to combat feelings of dehydration.

6. **What do I do if I'm still hungry? Do I eat more food or do I choose another snack?**

    You may have another snack. Simply refer to the snack section of this book for healthy snacking options. The premise for this 30~Day Detox is to lessen the load on your digestion, not to deprive you from food!

7. **If I exercise or workout a lot, can I have extra protein?**

    If it's needed, then add the extra protein, but make sure that you're getting the protein that your body needs to be able to detox properly the unwanted toxins from your body while still maintaining your active lifestyle. Please see the clean protein section of this book and add 3-4 ounces of good quality protein to each meal for a woman and 5 – 6 ounces for a man. I cannot stress enough that cleansing is not about deprivation!

    If you need more food, add a snack or more protein. Some people thrive better on an all raw, vegan, or vegetarian program while others need extra protein from animal sources, such as paleo or primal eating. We are all uniquely different beings based on our genes, stress and activity levels adding another snack or protein doesn't mean you're not succeeding at your detox, instead it

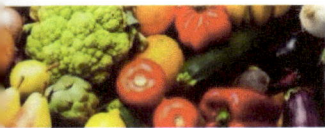

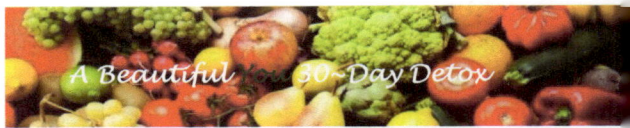

means that you are listening to your body and nourishing it with what it needs, the right way. You're doing it! So go ahead, throw in those few extra nuts!

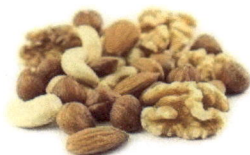

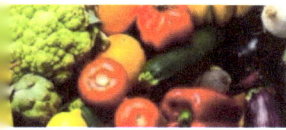

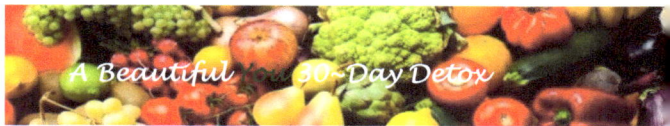

Chapter 4 – Probiotics and Cultured Foods

The What & How of Probiotics

Have you ever wondered where the word probiotic comes from and what it means? It's a copulation of two Greek words: "pro" meaning the promotion of and "biotic", life. All in all, it means "FOR LIFE"! You get the essentials of life from probiotics: good bacteria. If you take a good quality probiotic in liquid form or a capsule, or eating kefir, sauerkraut and other probiotic rich foods, you're effectively "crowding out" or replacing the bad bacteria with the good.

You may have never even thought about your digestive system as being directly related to achieving your weight loss goals, but you can bet that it is! There's a direct link associated with weight loss dealing with the balance of good bacteria in your intestines. Good bacteria is very important for a productive detox, proper digestion as well as a healthy immune system. Did you know that 75 to 80% of your immune system is in your digestive tract? So having good bacteria in your belly is a major preventative measure against things like the common cold, flue acid reflux, upset tummy (digestive upset), weight gain, allergies, sinus problems and arthritis and joint pain. Having the right amounts of good bacteria, you promote beautiful, glowing skin, a good and healthy weight and you'll feel fantabulous! This does not have to be a temporary fix! By changing your lifestyle, this can last a lifetime! When you balance the good bacteria in your gut, the weight melts off of you, you'll become acclimated with the changes that your body is going through and you'll leave all of the nasty side effects of a toxic body behind.

There's other great benefits of adding probiotics to regulate your bacteria…your bowels will move more frequently! Yep, you guessed it, POOHING! You can't hold it in and that's just a fact of life. If you're not going 1-3 times a day, then toxins that you've been trying to remove or that you've just removed will begin to build up in your colon again. This putrefied food then becomes an ideal breeding ground for bad bacteria, yeast and fungus. This is really bad as it contributes to weight gain, belly bloat, headaches, depression, sugar cravings and an unbalanced emotional state!

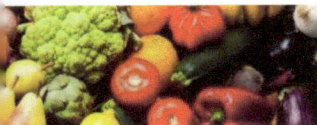

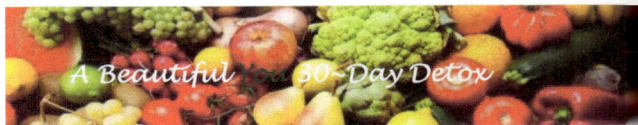

If at all you should become constipated on the Detox Program, which can happen, try using flaxseeds in a nighttime tea. You may want to drink a glass of it during the day also, or try organic herbal laxative tea. I put 1 tbsp. whole flaxseeds in a cup and pour water that's 118° and let it stand for about 45 minutes. Afterwards, drain the seeds and discard. Please be aware that not all people are the same as some folks will experience constipation on the Detox. It's a normal occurrence but will be alleviated by following the directions in this book.

These are some of the super powers that probiotics have:

- Improvement in digestive functions
- Improvement in liver function
- Decreases your toxicity levels
- Decreases your allergies
- Improves functions in the adrenals
- Increases your energy levels
- Sleep is improved
- Decreases or eliminates your acid reflux
- Helps get rid of or decreases bloating and gas
- Nutrients and minerals absorption is improved

Each and every day, you should want to add a great source of healthy bacteria to your body to improve digestion and affect better weight loss. Keep in mind that healthy weight loss begins with healthy digestion and is effortless. If your focus on this 30~Day Detox Program is to lessen food allergies, improve the equality of your skin, or just to really discover what foods work for your unique body, then probiotics is key. The best way to achieve this goal is to add at least one of these foods to your diet. Why not start with Good Belly drink or Dairy Free Bio-Kult (these are both natural foods and food based probiotics that can be found in most national grocery stores).

As Well As Cultured Foods

Cultured foods are another great source of probiotics. Cultured (fermented) foods will bring your body back into balance by giving you back your life. Good cultured foods include coconut water kefir, cultured veggies, miso soup, and kombucha.

Try consuming cultured foods with your meals to enhance your digestion, remove unwanted waste from the intestines and boost your immunity. You can find a lot of these

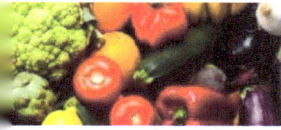

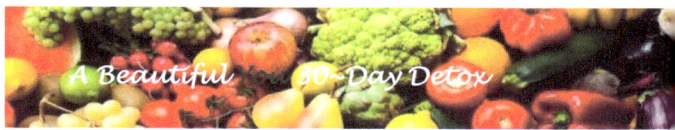

cultured foods at large grocery stores and whole foods stores. To start, do 2 tbsp. of cultured foods per meal, slowly work your way up to ¼ cup per meal. But keep in mind to be cautious when adding these probiotic foods to your meals. If you start out with too much, it can cause bloating, so start with only 2 tbsp. and increase gradually. Why not make it fun by preparing your own at home by using vegetables!

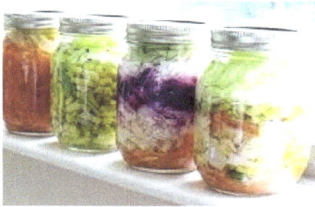

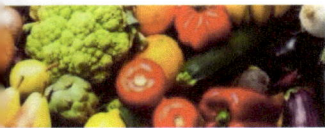

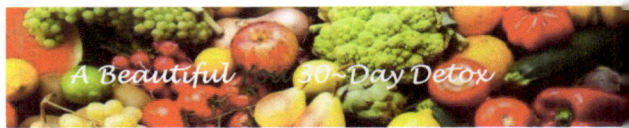

Chapter 5 – Get a Better Understanding of the Elimination Diet

How often do you listen to your own body when deciding what to eat, instead of listening to the media reports on what foods are supposed to be the best new foods? Some 10 years back, margarine was the best thing since sliced bread, now we see that butter is back. Take eggs for example, one day they're good for you, the next they're bad, then they're good again. How can one keep up? Cookie cutter nutrition guidance is problematic because some foods may not be good for your unique body. Have you ever thought of getting back to basics and listening to your own body? If not, why? You can do this by getting in tuned with your own body by listening to it and hearing what it's telling you. Your body is your personal engine…why not fine tune it. The elimination diet is the key to achieving a lifelong, healthy weight maintenance, healthy digestion and ditching dieting forever!

By doing the Elimination Diet and Detoxing, this gives you the opportunity to find out what really works for YOU personally. You will discover what actually fuels your engine properly. You will discover which foods sneakily wreaks havoc on your body and digestive system. Always keep in mind that by the end of this program, you will be running as efficiently as a racecar!

Pre-Tox Instructions

This stage is crucial because this is the stage that prepares the body for the changes that's about to occur for the betterment of your health. Crash detoxing can be harmful to the body if not done correctly and that is why during your Pre-Tox, you'll start to reduce or eliminate foods from the Elimination List. These foods causes all common allergens that's unrecognizable to many people. This leads to inflammation, followed by an increased toxicity in your body. During these 4 imperative days, you'll begin to reduce and get rid of these foods to prepare your body for the Detox and also help avoid the detox "I'm not feeling so good" syndrome! The "I'm not feeling so good" can occur when you remove foods that you usually consume and that tends to inflame your body. If you experience a headache after you stop consuming your favorite cereal or even your "Healthy "snack, not to worry as this is a good sign that you are uncovering what is not doing your body justice.

Food that you'll be eliminating are things like corn, grain, soy eggs, nuts sugar animal protein and sugar. The foods on the Elimination List are all commonly known to cause

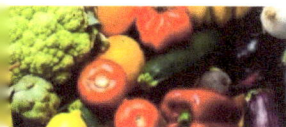

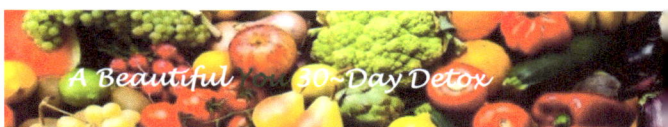

allergies, food sensitivities, moodiness, hormonal issues, digestive problems, inflammation and believe it or not, infertility! When you get rid of these foods, you give your digestive system a rest and you will automatically begin cleansing on a cellular level.

Detox Instructions

After you've done the Pre-Tox stage, you're now ready for the Detox stage. Set out for you in this book is a specific meal plan that you'll be following for the next 26 days. This will cleanse your body of the unwanted toxins and stress. I hope that you're as excited as I am for you! This is a journey that I know and/or hope you'll enjoy. Make sure you keep your journal and do your Feel Good Detoxing! Let the fun begin now!

Detox Transition Instructions

OK, so you've completed the 26 days of your detox! Now it's time to begin your 4 day Transition Stage. This stage is important, because this is the stage where you begin to reintroduce the foods on the Elimination List back into your diet one at a time, every two to three days. It's very important that you follow this to the letter to allow for a period of time to take note of any reactions, notice mood swings, and check for any inflammation that occurs when the body releases histamines. These histamines are released as a natural defense in the body. The body treats certain foods as allergens or other sensitivities that may occur. Your body responds to histamines in a negative reaction, WATER RETENTION!

This 30~Day Detox Program is your chance to look for any noticeable imbalances such as any mood changes, tummy gurgling, gas, bloating, constipation, weight gain and sleepless nights. All of these symptoms are signs of imbalances and what I suggest is for you to wait 5 – 7 days to reintroduce a food if you notice any of these reactions after you reintroduce any foods from the Elimination List. During this process, you'll really learn what foods causes you to have inflammation and the ones that gives you vibrant energy. In the recipe section of this book, you find a Transitional Recipe Section. Please refer to the recipes to guide you along the way for those remaining four days and try adding foods back into your diet after the Detox Program.

As I mentioned earlier, keep a journal of any and all food reactions and your overall experience. This is a wonderful way to get in tuned with your body. Just keep in mind that finding the right foods for your body equals weight loss and lifelong, easy maintenance!

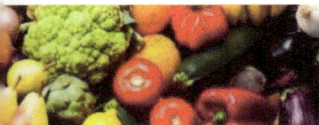

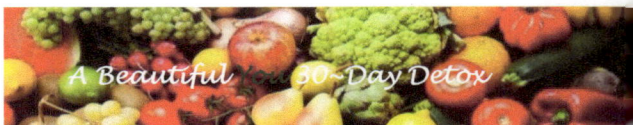

The Elimination Diet is the premise for your success. Your body never stays the same and is changing day-by-day, and year-to-year and yes season to season! You may have noticed that a diet that you tried years ago, may not work for you today. It's important that you take time throughout the year to go through this process and get your body back in shape!

Your Food Journal – Writing It All Down

Beginning with the day of your Pre-Tox, start journaling. Write down how your feeling, are you anxious, nervous, are you having headaches, nausea. You will be provided a food journal in this book. Please put this form to good use by making it a habit of keeping up with your meals, mood and how you're doing overall. You will be doing this before, after and during each meal, snack and beverage. At first, you may feel odd or may not feel effects from it at all. That's ok too because you may find at times you're simply jotting down that you feel "good" or "fine". Other times, there may be more to your account.

Journaling is designed to be a fun process for you. It's a great tool because it allows you a moment for clarity on your day, your body's results and how your Detox is coming along. As you move forward, your journaling will serve as your own little research guide as to what works for you and what doesn't and will help keep you on the right path for success. This is your chance to finally determine what works for your body. Once you learn what foods are right for you, easy weight loss, radiant skin and feeling and looking 10-15 years younger are all in your power.

Listed are a few examples to put you on the right path for your journaling. Please refer to your Journal and Big Picture Vision section of this book for help in this area.

Physical Sensations of Your Body

- Symptoms of imbalances: headaches, pain in your stomach, muscle or leg cramps, constant coughing, fatigue, insomnia, shakiness, restlessness, muscle weakness, paleness, trouble concentrating
- Symptoms of balance: bright eyed, hunger, vigor, breathing deeply naturally, highly energetic, well rested, good quality sleep, awareness, strength, good attention span, good color

Page | 29

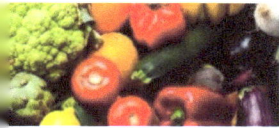

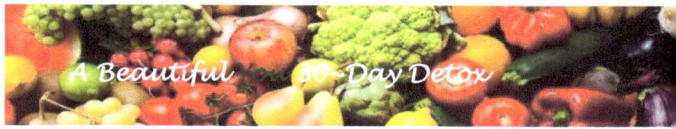

Your Emotions May Be More Difficult to Gage

- Symptoms of imbalances: anxious, bored, scared mad, sad, depressed, unfocused, restless, easily irritated, stressed, wired, twitchy
- Symptoms of balance: self-assured, enthusiastic, eager, amusing, happy, attentive, motivated, tranquil, relaxed, serene, enduring

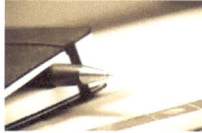

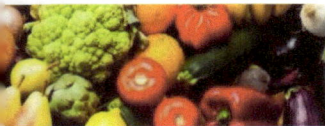

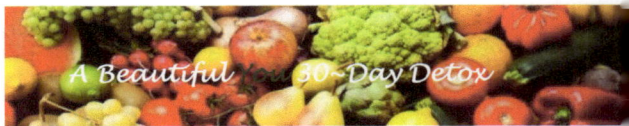

Chapter 6 – What Level Are You?

When it comes to your comfort zone, only you know your level when it comes to detoxing and cleansing your body. Even though it always helps to lessen unwanted detox symptoms, do not stay at the same detox level while on this program. Start by identifying the level below that best defines you.

1. Begin at level 1 if:
    - You're a newbie to cleansing and detoxing
    - You're at a stage where you're eating pasta, bread and processed foods
    - You're now eating a couple of servings of dairy on a daily basis, any dairy
    - You're eating a large amount of sugar
    - You have 4 or more cups of coffee a day
    - You don't feel comfortable with the phrase "Detox"

2. Begin at level 2 if:
    - You've done a detox before
    - You eat bread, pasta, sugar or processed foods only on occasion
    - You're currently eating fresh fruits, veggies and whole foods on a daily basis
    - You're currently drinking green smoothies or have tried juicing in the past

3. Begin at level 3 if:
    - You're not at all afraid of doing a detox easily
    - You're already eating greens, fruits and whole foods on a daily basis
    - You're ready to take this challenge and just go for it

This 30~Day Detox Program is broken down into three stages and within those three groups, I'm personalizing this Detox Program even further for you.

If you're only at Level 1:

- Please go over the FAQ's again to get the sense of the Detox as well as the weight loss process.
- Try and eliminate the sugar in your diet and get rid of the processed foods during the Pre-Tox stage. Begin to drink the Lemon/Lime Water Regimen at

Page | 31

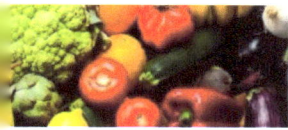

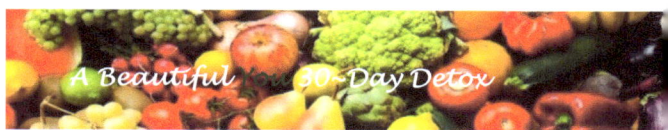

the start of the day upon rising. It is ok if you need a couple (2) cups of coffee in your daily routine at this point. The coffee habit can be a tough one to break as you can suffer withdrawal, so take the time to reduce it slowly by ¼ cup per day or just drink one cop of organic coffee during your Detox.

- Remember, stay HYDRATED to avoid an upset tummy, constipation as well as nausea.

- If you think that you'll need an extra snack during the 26 Detox days, just go to the Snack Section of this book. Do not buy snacks pre-packaged from the grocery store as this will set you back and possible upset your stomach.

- If you feel like things are happening too fast on the Detox and you begin to feel strong symptoms of detoxing, like nausea, then take it down a notch. Add a cup of brown rice, quinoa or gluten free oatmeal with some almond, coconut or rice milk and a pinch of stevia. Also try a banana with a little tahini or some gluten free bread with almond-butter and honey. Be aware that this may slow your weight loss goals, but again detoxing is about feeling light, happy and fancy free. I don't want you to feel stressed out or overly uncomfortable.

- Be aware of how you're feeling. Be sure that you're getting enough protein with every meal. Too little protein will make you feel nauseated. If you feel it necessary to add 4 ounces of fish or ¼ cup of beans, or an extra vegetarian protein options to your meal, then please refer to the Elimination List and choose beans that are approved during your Detox.

- You also need to be aware of the fact that you can begin to feel feelings of sadness or being overly emotional during your detox. Anger may rear its ugly head also. Detoxing can bring out many emotions, so when this happens, just remain calm and know that this is a symptom of your body detoxing and getting rid of unwanted toxins from your body. Just remember, those negative feelings that you're experiencing, they'll be released as well, just let them go.

If you're at Level 2:

- Follow the Detox Program step by step and pay attention to what your body's telling you. If you need an extra snack, just refer to the Snack Section in this book.

- You may be familiar with detoxing especially if you've done it before and therefore realize that it's not just physical, but also emotional as well. To circumvent any physical Detox "I'm not feeling so good" symptoms, please begin doing the Detox "Feeling Great" during the Pre-Tox.

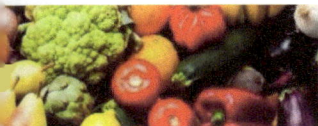

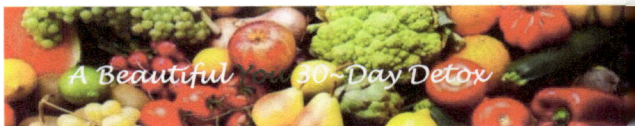

↓ You can also follow the suggestions for the Level 3 Detox Genius!

If you're at Level 3:

↓ You may add juices (ones that you've juiced yourself) to your daily detoxing to alkalize and support optimal detox and weight loss. You can have it upon rising in the morning or add it to a snack in the afternoon, or as a pick-me-up. You can do a 1 day juice fast with extra snacks, plan on doing this while doing the Pre-Tox. Choose 3 juices to use for the day and consume 4 ounces of coconut water for snacks with ½ cup unsweetened fruit like berries for a little extra nutrition. If you feel that you need a little more just to get you going, then add a tbsp. coconut oil with each glass of juice.

↓ Keep in mind that even the healthiest eaters and the more experienced Detox Geniuses still have a measure of toxicity in their bodies, so enjoy your journey and get rid of the baggage that's not serving your purpose.

So, set your fears aside and kiss your toxic body goodbye!

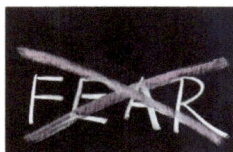

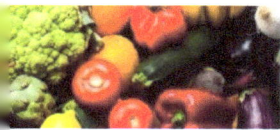

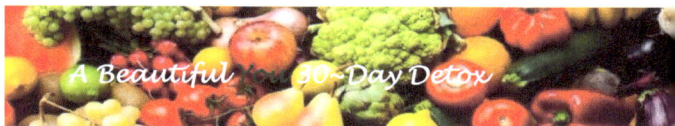

Chapter 7 – Making Preparations & Planning For Your Detox

This is how the Spectacular You: 30~Day Detox Program is arranged for your benefit:

Pre-Tox: Preparation for the Elimination Diet (4 days)

Detox: Tactical Elimination Diet (26 days)

Transition Diet: Transition to Clean Eating (4 days)

How to Prep

The first and far most part of the Detox is your preparation or pre-start and pre-planning. It is a crucial step leading to your success on this plan. The more you prepare, the less stressed you'll feel during the program about what or/and when to eat. THIS STEP IS KEY FOR AN ENJOYABLE DETOX! Look for more helpful tips on this matter by referring to the Staging Your Kitchen section in this book.

1. Peruse through the meal plan section of this book to familiarize yourself with the step-by-step what and when to eat for the next 30 days (26 days Detox and 4 days Transition). Look over the Recipe Section and begin taking note of the meals you would like to include in your personal Detox. Keep in mind that it's important not to choose Recipes from the Transition Section during your Detox Stage. Transition Recipe are clearly marked at the end of the Recipe Section in this book.
2. Once you've decided on your selection, use the Meal Planner to document your meal choices if they differ from the meals provided for you in the 30 day meal planner.
3. Make sure to use the shopping list provided you to mark off the ingredients that you'll need for your menu.

The Pre-Tox

For the first 4 days of the 30~Day Detox Program, you'll be focusing on the pre-prepping part of the Detox. Always keep in mind that this Detox is all about eliminating foods that may be causing your body unwanted bloat, inflammation and weight gain and is keeping

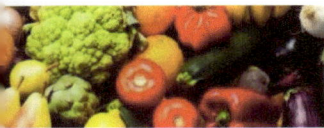

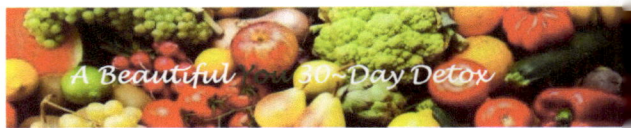

you from feeling and looking fantabulous. Using the Elimination List, you'll begin reducing foods that are not included in the Detox. This Pre-Tox course helps to reduce and avoid some of the more common symptoms of Detoxing you might go through during the actual Detox Stage, such as headaches, moodiness and tiredness. Pre-Toxing can even set your body in the Detox mode and therefore initiate detox symptoms, so look to your Detox "feeling great" in this book to start doing them now. As I mentioned before, you can also begin to drink your Lemon or Lime Water Regimen every morning during Pre-Tox.

Elimination List

Begin reducing and eliminating these foods during your Pre-Tox:

- Caffeine – if you drink coffee, slowly reduce your consumption by ¼ cup daily. Remember, if you want to continue drinking coffee during your Detox, only drink one cup of organic coffee each morning. You may also consider switching to dandelion coffee, or decaffeinated green tea. These items can be found at your local Whole Foods Market.
- Eliminate white sugar and replace it with either raw honey or stevia in the raw
- Processed foods
- Gluten
- Grains
- Nuts
- Alcohol
- Soy, with the exception of miso past and wheat free tamari (do not use if intolerant).
- Dairy
- Beans (begin by reducing hard to digest beans during the Pre-Tox stage. Beans that you may have during the Detox stage include mung, lentils and adzuki, as they are easily digested.)

Successful Detox Tips

- **Clean out your fridge and cupboards:** Get rid of foods that may tempt you. What for? Because we are setting the stage for an amazing weight loss & a superb Detoxing. If you have to give it all away, I don't care, you can even donate it. And most importantly, DO NOT BINGE on the foods that's in your fridge or cupboards just to get rid of it.
- **Goals: Set your personal goals and right them down NOW!:** Take the time to write down your goals in your journal or use a sticky note and post it up in

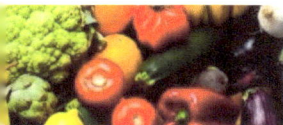

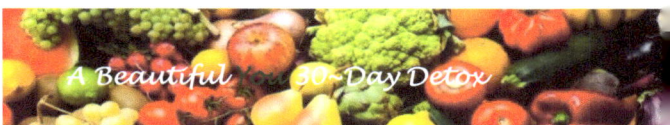

your bedroom and/or bedroom mirror to remind you of it every day. In this way if you put it there, you'll see it.

- **Get a buddy to detox with or corral your family!** Make sure that your family is on the same page that you're on. You don't need any sabotagers getting in the way of your Detox Program. Let them know that you're kicking the junk food habit and replacing them with healing foods that's going to get you going to a healthier, happier life!

- **Your Time!** Means just that! Taking the time out for yourself. Decide on an activity every day that you will add during your Detox to honor yourself and set yourself up for true success.

Always Remember – "Live More, Stress Less & Weigh Less"

Before you scheduled "you time", say these words to yourself every day!

The Emotional Facets of Detoxing and Weight Loss

It's very important that you don't think of a detox and weight loss as simply a physical experience. Weight loss is certainly not just about the food on your plate.

Begin doing a daily journal not only about your relationship with food, but also the relationships you may have with other people included in your life. Many times, we eat when we are sad, depressed, tired and stressed or just depleted. Some people may go through these feelings during detoxing because they haven't learned how to create for themselves "YES & NO" boundaries; please develop perfect boundaries and develop the art of saying "NO!"

Can you count the times where you found yourself saying yes when deep down in your heart and soul, your gut feeling is screaming NO? Do you also find that you're putting yourself at the bottom of the Totem Pole, sacrificing your healthy eating, exercise and quiet time?

TIME TO GET CREATIVE! FIND THAT NECESSARY "YOU TIME" BY PUTTING YOU FIRST!

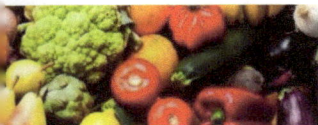

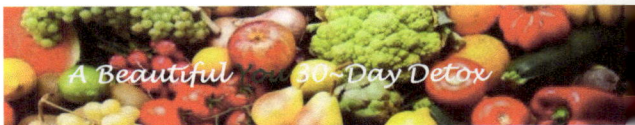

Journal Exercise: Write about your feelings coming up for you during this Detox. Look for the common ones like sadness, anger as well as resentment. All though you can't change some of the behaviors right away, journaling will at least give you the chance to review your patterns. This is also useful in pointing out those activities and people in your day that are only depleting you and not providing any positive feedback in return. This goes hand in hand with your homework to journal your intention for the day every morning and evening to get retrospect on your emotions that for that day. This record will be a great tool for you moving towards your post detox.

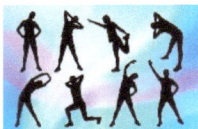

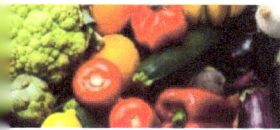

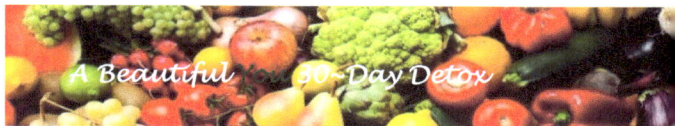

Chapter 8 - The Daily To-Do List for Detoxing

Please complete these daily tasks to fully support your liver functions, lessen any unwanted detox symptoms and help aid easier weight loss:

- o Brush your tongue – cleaning your tongue every morning and evening promotes optimal detoxing: When using the rounded edge of a tongue scraper, gently scrape down the tongue several times while applying gentle pressure. Rinse the tongue scraper under running water and gently repeat this process again until there's no white residue left on the tongue. Try doing this 2 – 3 times daily or after you brush your teeth.
- o Drink your Lemon/Lime Regimen.
- o Take your probiotic to add good bacteria to your gut. (optional)
- o Do your journal. Write down your goals for the day in the morning and your reflection of the day that night.
- o Before you begin your Transition Stage, create your Big Picture Vision.
- o Do a Daily Meditation: Focus on your prayers to God and put the negative thoughts out of your mind. Do deep breathing as you meditate to on your prayers. This helps to eliminate the negative energies that's within your body. Take deep breathes in and exhale out the toxins and the negativities! When you breathe in, hold this breath as long as you can, visualize peace and do this for 10 minutes per day. Think about the oxygen flowing in through your nostrils, promoting good health all the way down to your toes and as you exhale, release the old and when you inhale, take in the good. Keep in mind, we do our best breathing when we're relaxed, so put on some soothing music, in my case, Kingdom Melodies, and find a comforting place where you can become relaxed. Close your eyes and let go of all toxins, anger, sadness and any other emotions that you may be holding on to with a negative attachment.
- o Do your regular workouts, sit in a sauna, or jump on a mini trampoline, move your body to release the endorphins and get your body sweating. Sweating is a crucial element of detoxing.
- o Refer to your Detox Feeling Greats to decrease any unwanted detox symptoms. Remember, these activities are wonderful Pre-Tox, Detox and Transition AND for the rest of your life!

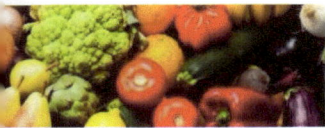

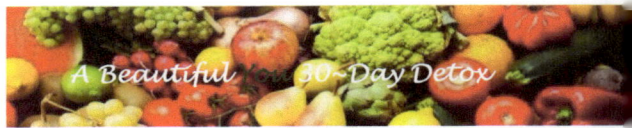

Have Fun Planning Your Meals

Protein During Your Detox

There's no right or wrong during a detox. Everyone is different! Some of us need more protein to invigorate, rebuild cell, detox the right way and think clearly. LISTEN to your body!

You're permitted to add 3 – 4 ounces of a clean protein source to any meal if needed.

Sources of Clean Protein:

* **Beans** (Mung, Adzuki)
* **Lentils**
* **Seeds** (Hemp, Sunflower, Pumpkin, Pea Protein Powder)

Juicing While Detoxing

The Recipe Section of this book contains a few great recipes – Liquid Gold. If you have a juicer, I recommend drinking a juice daily as your breakfast or afternoon snack in order to get your body to an alkalized state. The more alkalized your body, the less chances for unwanted diseases. These juice recipes are designed to detox your body on a cellular level. If you don't have a juicer, you'll still be able to follow the meal plan and complete your detox very successfully!

Your Daily Drinking Guide

Drinking to Flush Out the Toxins

Morning Lemon / Lime Regimen
1 10 oz. glass of warm water
Juice from ½ lemon and ½ lime (approximately 1 tbsp. each)
1/10 tsp. tabasco or cayenne pepper (or half of 1/8 tsp)
2 tbsp. pure maple syrup
~This stimulates digestion, releases toxins from the liver and jump-starts your digestive enzymes.

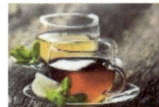

Midday Cranberry Cleansing Flush
2 tbsp. cranberry concentrate (Knudsen's is the best if you can find it at your local grocers)
6 ounces room temp water (feel free to add stevia to sweeten the pot a little)
~Great as a flush for the lymphatic system, cleansing unwanted bacteria, detoxing & weight loss)

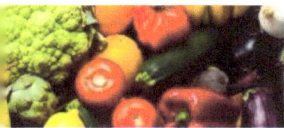

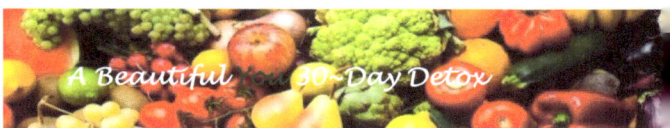

Coconut Water Kefir or Plain Coconut Water

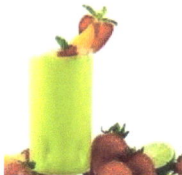

Consume 4 ounces of coconut water or 2 ounces of coconut water kefir between breakfast and lunch. Take caution that your coconut water has no added sugar. When it doubt, fresh is best, but if you can't find fresh the commercial brand Zico is a good option. Also try a raw coconut drink! It's a fabulous choice, but can be more expensive!

For healthy seasonal recipes, please visit www.holisticlifestylechanges.com and get recipes for the change of seasons!

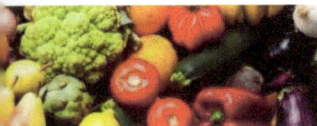

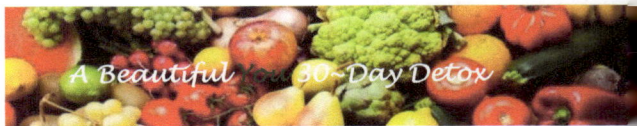

Chapter 9 – Your Detox Program

Your Detox Success Depends on Your Commitment to Your Elimination Diet as well as Your Transition Diet

Reminder: If you're on a tight schedule, then don't worry about the time allotments in this schedule as these are only suggested times only. I want you to de-stress, not be stressed. Feel free to adjust the times to your busy schedule. This program is also flexible as you can exchange recipes or add extra protein to each meal (Choose from the Clean Plant Based Proteins area of this book).

Reminder: For seasonal fruits and veggies detox recipes, please visit www.holisticlifestlechanges.com on the recipe page and get seasonal detox recipes to fit the season!

Reminder: If you possess a juicer, then please juice every day in the morning or use as a snack at 11:30 AM or 4:00 PM and add to coconut water to add essential minerals.

* Or when you're up in the morning or if your work nights.

Day One
- 7:00 am * Morning Lemon / Lime Regimen with Probiotic
- 8:00 am herbal tea or organic coffee
- 10:00 am **Breakfast**: Sassy Raw Smoothie
- 11:30 am Coconut Water (4 ounces), add if a Snack is desired
- 1:30 pm **Lunch**: Orange Arugula Salad
- 4:00 pm **Snack**: 2 tablespoons Detoxing Pesto with Raw Veggies, Cranberry Cleansing Flush.
- 6:00 pm **Dinner**: Curried Butternut Squash with Broccoli

Day Two
- 7:00 am * Morning Lemon / Lime Regimen with Probiotic
- 8:00 am herbal tea or organic coffee
- 10:00 am **Breakfast**: Thunderbolt With a Dash of Sunshine Smoothie
- 11:00 am Coconut Water (4 ounces) add a snack if desired

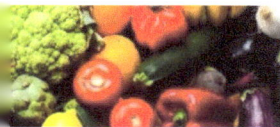

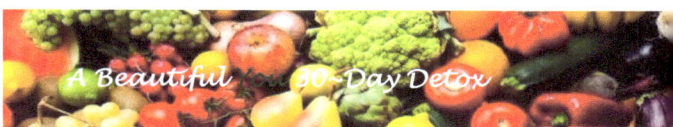

- 1:30 pm **Lunch**: Detox Your Body Lettuce Wraps
- 4:00 pm **Snack**: 2 tbsp. Detoxing Pesto with Raw Veggies, along with Cleansing Flush
- 6:00 pm **Dinner**: Coconut Brussels Sprouts and Beets

Day Three

- 7:00 am * Morning Lemon / Lime Regimen with Probiotic
- 8:00 am herbal tea or organic coffee
- 10:00 am **Breakfast**: Black & Strawberry Dreamsicle Smoothie
- 11:30 am Coconut Water (4 ounces) add a snack if needed
- 1:30 pm **Lunch**: Dijon Corn Salad
- 4:00 pm **Snack**: Mexicali Dip with Raw Veggies, Cleansing Flush
- 600 pm **Dinner**: Cream of Cauliflower Soup

Day Four

- 7:00 am * Morning Lemon / Lime Regimen with Probiotic
- 8:00 am herbal tea or one cup organic coffee
- 10:00 am **Breakfast**: Greased Lightning Smoothie
- 11:30 am Coconut Water (4 ounces) add snack if needed
- 1:30 pm **Lunch**: Sweet & Sexy Detox Salad
- 4:00 pm **Snack**: ½ avocado with 1 slice tomato & cucumber, seasoned with sea salt, pepper and garlic with Cleansing Flush
- 6:00 pm **Dinner**: Cream of Spinach Soup

Day Five

- 7:00 am * Morning Lemon / Lime Regimen with Probiotic
- 8:00 am herbal tea or one cup organic coffee
- 10:00 am **Breakfast**: Chocolate Covered Cherries Smoothie
- 11:30 am Coconut Water (4 ounces) add snack if needed
- 1:30 pm **Lunch**: Tomato Fennel Salad
- 4:00 pm **Snack**: ½ grapefruit sliced with unsweetened coconut topped with 2 tbsp. Tahini sprinkled with a little cinnamon, Cleansing Flush
- 6:00 **Dinner**: Confetti Rice

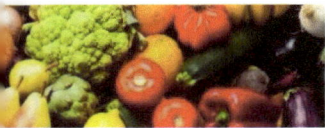

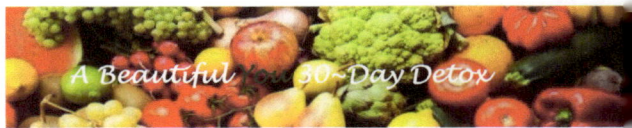

Day Six

- 7:00 am * Morning Lemon / Lime Regimen with Probiotic
- 8:00 am herbal tea or organic coffee
- 10:00 am **Breakfast**: Sleek & Sassy Smoothie
- 11:30 am Coconut Water (4 ounces) add snack if needed
- 1:30 pm **Lunch**: Lavish Berry Salad with Pineapple Ginger Dressing
- 4:00 pm **Snack**: Detoxing Pesto with ½ sweet potato, Cleansing Flush
- 6:00 pm **Dinner**: Healthy Bowl with Orange Zest

Day Seven

- 7:00 am * Morning Lemon / Lime Regimen with Probiotic
- 8:00 am herbal tea or organic coffee
- 10:00 am **Breakfast**: Sassy Raw Smoothie
- 11:30 am Coconut Water (4 ounces) add snack if needed
- 1:30 pm **Lunch**: Orange Arugula Salad
- 4:00 pm **Snack**: green apple (Granny Smith) with 2 tbsp. Tahini with Cleansing Flush
- 6:00 pm **Dinner**: Cream of Cauliflower Soup

Day Eight

- 7:00 am * Morning Lemon / Lime Regimen with Probiotic
- 8:00 am herbal tea or organic coffee
- 10:00 am **Breakfast**: Banana-Mango Tropics Smoothie
- 11:30 am Coconut Water (4 ounces) add snack if needed
- 1:30 pm **Lunch**: Mediterranean Style Kale Salad
- 4:00 pm **Snack**: Ants on a Log, Cleansing Flush
- 6:00 pm **Dinner**: Carrot Hazelnut Soup

Day Nine

- 7:00 am * Morning Lemon / Lime Regimen with Probiotic
- 8:00 am herbal tea or organic coffee
- 10:00 **Breakfast**: Orange-Cantaloupe Hit The Tropics Smoothie
- 11:30 am Coconut Water (4 ounces) add snack if needed
- 1:30 pm **Lunch**: A Raisin In The Sun Broccoli Salad
- 4:00 pm **Snack**: ½ avocado with 1 slice of tomato and cucumber, seasoned with sea salt pepper and garlic powder, Cleansing Flush
- 6:00 pm **Dinner**: Bok Choy, Coconut Soup

Page | 43

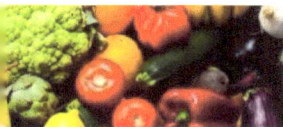

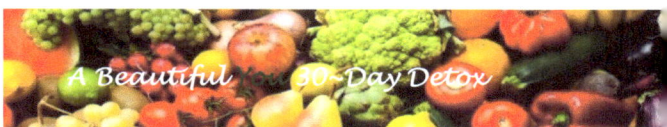

Day Ten

- 7:00 am * Morning Lemon / Lime Regimen with Probiotic
- 8:00 am herbal tea or organic coffee
- 10:00 am **Breakfast**: Banilla-Orange Smoothie
- 11:30 am Coconut Water (4 ounces) add snack if needed
- 1:30 pm **Lunch**: Sweet & Sour Cucumber Salad with Dill
- 4:00 pm **Snack**: Zucchini Steamboat, Cleansing Flush
- 6:00 pm **Dinner**: Raw Tomato Basil Soup

Day Eleven

- 7:00 am * Morning Lemon / Lime Regimen with Probiotic
- 8:00 am herbal tea or organic coffee
- 10:00 am **Breakfast**: Pineapple Orange Delight Smoothie
- 11:30 am Coconut Water (4 ounces) add snack if needed
- 1:30 pm **Lunch**: Cream of Asparagus Soup
- 4:00 pm **Snack**: Banana-Tahini Celery Delight
- 6:00 pm **Dinner**: Cress Salad with Golden Beets

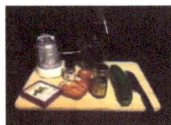

Day Twelve

- 7:00 am * Morning Lemon / Lime Regimen with Probiotic
- 8:00 am herbal tea or organic coffee
- 10:00 am **Breakfast**: Banana-Less Pineapple-Orange Smoothie
- 11:30 am Coconut Water (4 ounces) add snack if needed
- 1:30 pm **Lunch**: Raw Spaghetti with Raw Marinara Sauce
- 4:00 pm **Snack**: Scrumptious Poppers, Cleansing Flush
- 6:00 pm **Dinner**: Raw Roasted Tomato Soup

Day Thirteen

- 7:00 am * Morning Lemon / Lime Regimen
- 8:00 am herbal tea or organic coffee
- 10:00 am **Breakfast**: Orange Madness Smoothie
- 11:30 am Coconut Water (4 ounces) add a snack if needed
- 1:30 pm **Lunch**: Peachy Kale Salad with Miso Vinaigrette
- 4:00 pm **Snack**: Banana-Tahini Celery Delight, Cleansing Flush
- 6:00 pm **Dinner**: Healthy Bowl with Orange Zest

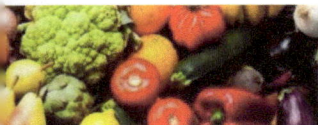

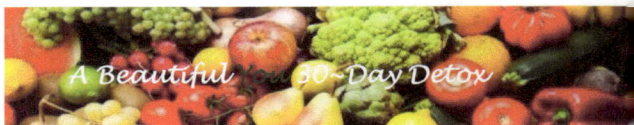

Day Fourteen

- 7:00 am * Morning Lemon / Lime Regimen
- 8:00 am herbal tea or organic coffee
- 10:00 am **Breakfast**: Vanilla-Pineapple Sunrise Smoothie
- 11:30 am Coconut Water (4 ounces) add snack if needed
- 1:30 pm **Lunch**: The Radish Has It Salad with Curry Vinaigrette
- 4:00 pm **Snack**: Lemony Cups, Cleansing Flush
- 6:00 pm **Dinner**: Confetti Rice

Day Fifteen

- 7:00 am * Morning Lemon / Lime Regimen
- 8:00 am herbal tea or organic coffee
- 10:00 am **Breakfast**: Mango Tango Smoothie
- 11:30 am Coconut Water (4 ounces) add snack if needed
- 1:30 pm **Lunch**: Jicama Salad with Smashing Curry Sauce
- 4:00 pm **Snack**: Raw Granola, Cleansing Flush
- 6:00 pm **Dinner**: Raw Butternut Squash Soup

Day Sixteen

- 7:00 am * Morning Lemon / Lime Regimen
- 8:00 am herbal tea or organic coffee
- 10:00 am **Breakfast**: Papapple Smoothie
- 11:30 am Coconut Water (4 ounces) add snack if needed
- 1:30 pm **Lunch**: Berry-Mango Salad
- 4:00 pm **Snack**: Ants on a Log, Cleansing Flush
- 6:00 pm **Dinner**: Cream of Spinach Soup

Day Seventeen

- 7:00 am * Morning Lemon / Lime Regime
- 8:00 am herbal tea or organic coffee
- 10:00 am **Breakfast**: Banana-Strawberry Smoothie
- 11:30 am Coconut Water (4 ounces) add snack if needed
- 1:30 pm **Lunch**: Luscious Melon Salad with Mint
- 4:00 pm **Snack**: Dilly Stuffed Tomatoes, Cleansing Flush
- 6:00 pm **Dinner**: Cream of Cauliflower Soup

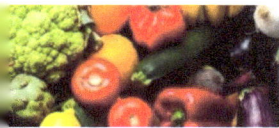

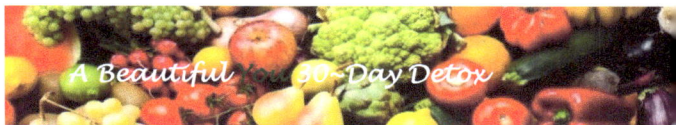

Day Eighteen

- 7:00 am * Morning Lemon / Lime Regimen
- 8:00 am herbal tea or organic coffee
- 10:00 am **Breakfast**: Simply Nourishing Smoothie
- 11:30 am Coconut Water (4 ounces) add snack if needed
- 1:30 pm **Lunch**: Heirloom Tomatoes with Mexi-Cali Salad
- 4:00 pm **Snack**: Dressed Up Zucchini with Veggies, Cleansing Flush
- 6:00 pm **Dinner**: Ginger Kale Soup with Miso

Day Nineteen

- 7:00 am * Morning Lemon / Lime Regimen
- 8:00 am herbal tea or organic coffee
- 10:00 am **Breakfast**: Great Day In The Morning Smoothie
- 11:30 am Coconut Water (4 ounces) add snack if needed
- 1:30 pm **Lunch**: Vietnamese Pho Soup
- 4:00 pm **Snack**: Tea Sandwiches in the Raw, Cleansing Flush
- 6:00 pm **Dinner**: Hot "N" Spicy Bok Choy Soup

Day Twenty

- 7:00 am * Morning Lemon / Lime Regimen
- 8:00 am herbal tea or organic coffee
- 10:00 am **Breakfast**: Peachy Keen Smoothie
- 11:30 am Coconut Water (4 ounces) add snack if needed
- 1:30 pm **Lunch**: Luscious Summer Salad
- 4:00 pm **Snack**: 2 tbsp. Detoxing Pesto with ½ sweet potato, Cleansing Flush
- 6:00 pm **Dinner**: Curried Butternut Squash with Broccoli

Day Twenty-One

- 7:00 am * Morning Lemon / Lime Regimen
- 8:00 am herbal tea or organic coffee
- 10:00 am **Breakfast**: Smoothie with a Kick
- 11:30 am **Coconut** Water (4 ounces) add snack if needed
- 1:30 pm **Lunch**: Dancing on the Tongue Slaw
- 4:00 pm **Snack**: Collard Wrap, Cleansing Flush
- 6:00 pm **Dinner**: Red Romaine Tomato Cucumber Salad

Day Twenty-Two

- 7:00 am * Morning Lemon / Lime Regimen
- 8:00 am herbal tea or organic coffee
- 10:00 am **Breakfast**: Avocado Delight Smoothie
- 11:30 am Coconut Water (4 ounces) add snack if needed
- 1:30 pm **Lunch**: Sun Dried Tomato Spread Dressed in Green
- 4:00 pm **Snack**: ½ Grapefruit sliced with 2 tbsp. unsweetened coconut with 2 tbsp. Tahini with a dash of cinnamon, Cleansing Flush
- 6:00 pm **Dinner**: Tomato Basil Soup

Day Twenty-Three

- 7:00 am * Morning Lemon / Lime Regimen
- 8:00 am herbal tea or organic coffee
- 10:00 am **Breakfast**: Happy Cucumber "N" Melon Smoothie
- 11:30 am Coconut Water (4 ounces) add snack if needed
- 1:30 pm **Lunch**: Lavish Berry Salad
- 4:00 pm **Snack**: ½ Avocado with 1 Slice Tomato & Cucumber, seasoned with sea salt, pepper, and garlic powder, Cleansing Flush
- 6:00 pm **Dinner**: Creamy Spinach Soup

Day Twenty-Four

- 7:00 am * Morning Lemon / Lime Regimen
- 8:00 am herbal tea or organic coffee
- 10:00 am **Breakfast**: Cantaloupe Delight Smoothie
- 11:30 am Coconut Water (4 ounces) add snack if needed
- 1:30 pm **Lunch**: Carrot Curry Salad
- 4:00 pm **Snack**: Banana-Tahini Celery Delight, Cleansing Flush
- 6:00 pm **Dinner**: Curried Broccoli with Butternut Squash

Day Twenty-Five

- 7:00 am * Morning Lemon / Lime Regimen
- 8:00 am herbal tea or organic coffee
- 10:00 am **Breakfast**: Carrot-Apricot Delight Smoothie
- 11:30 am Coconut Water (4 ounces) add snack if needed
- 1:30 pm **Lunch**: Creamy Carrot Soup
- 4:00 pm **Snack**: Green Apple with 2 tbsp. Tahini, Cleansing Flush
- 6:00 pm **Dinner**: Mediterranean Style Kale Salad

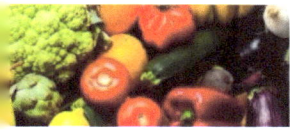

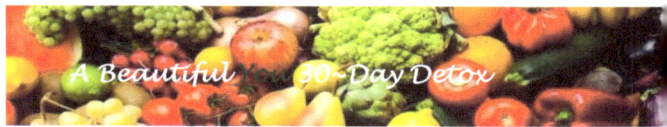

Day Twenty-Six

- 7:00 am * Morning Lemon / Lime Regimen
- 8:00 am herbal tea or organic coffee
- 10:00 am **Breakfast**: Fruity Zucchini Smoothie
- 11:30 am Coconut Water (4 ounces) add snack if needed
- 1:30 pm **Lunch**: Marinated Cucumbers
- 4:00 pm **Snack**: Ants on a Log, Cleansing Flush
- 6:00 pm **Dinner**: Tomato Gazpacho (Gluten Free)

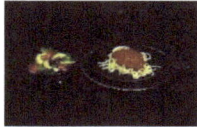

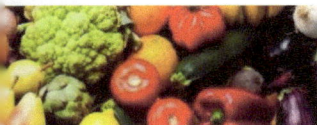

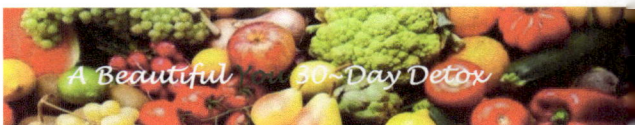

Chapter 10 – Your Transition

CONGRATULATIONS! Are you as excited as I am? You should be, because you've just completed 26 days of your Elimination Diet. Now, you're going to begin the next stage of your program, the Transition Stage. For the next 4 days, you'll begin slowly adding in foods from the Elimination List back into your diet, a little at a time or one food at a time. Please remember to keep journaling during this Transition Stage. This is a crucial step that you don't want to cease doing as this is your chance to really discover what foods ae right for your unique body. As I mentioned earlier, often an inability to lose weight is connected to inflammation caused by eating foods that your body cannot tolerate. This Transition Stage is your opportunity to get the sense of what's creating inflammation in your body so that you can more easily and effectively decrease the inflammation, lose weight and ditch dieting forever!

But before you go any further, create your Big Picture Vision. This is going to help make all of your goals such a reality that'll last a lifetime. Don't forget, review the Journaling and Big Picture Vision section in this book for more on this topic.

Your Food Diary

Your Food Diary is a very powerful tool. Taking advantage of the Food Diary provides you with a brand new perspective on how foods affect you both physically and emotionally. Feel free to use the form in this book or you can create your own…it's just easier to use the one in the book as you'll be using your book on a daily basis. Make notes on how you feel emotionally as well as physically, before, during and after each meal, snack and beverage. For example, by now, you should know how fantabulous it feels not to be bloated, so notice if that sensation returns when you add foods back in from the Elimination List or that wasn't on your Detox menu.

Examples:

> ➢ Are you tired?
> ➢ Are you bloated?
> ➢ Are you irritated
> ➢ Are you having pain in your lower back?
> ➢ Are you constipated?

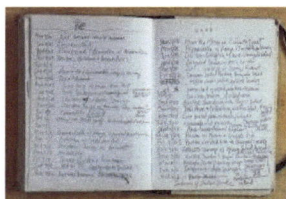

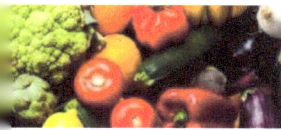

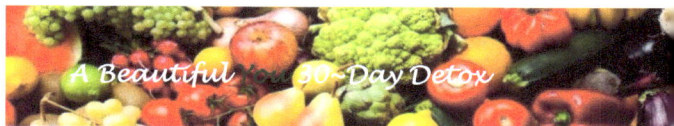

This is a crucial stage! So get excited! Here's your chance to finally ditch all diets that don't work and stop counting calories with no need to dwell on carbs, proteins or fats. We need to be focusing on the foods that's keeping you feeling and looking fantastic every second of the day, nothing else matters!

The Transition Stage of your Fantastic You: 30~Day Detox Program should be the most fun and informative as well. Keep telling yourself that no food is generally good or bad. Your relationship with food should only be defined by what fuels your body, giving you endless energy, and what causes inflammation in you.

Just a little reminder of the reactions and symptoms. These examples are to keep you motivated and on target:

Physical Sensations of Your Body

- Symptoms of imbalance: headaches, stomach upset, muscle cramps, constant coughing, tiredness, insomnia, sleeplessness, shakiness muscle weakness, lack of concentration, paleness
- Symptoms of balance: bright eyed, satiety, vigor, natural deep breathing, energetic restful, good sleep, focused alertness, stamina, good attention span, great color

Your Emotions May Be More Difficult To Gage

- Symptoms of imbalance: anxiety, bored, scared, angry, sad, depressed, unfocused, restless, irritated, agitated, wired
- Symptoms of balance: confident, excited, energetic, gregarious, happy interested, focused, calm, relaxed, easygoing, patient.

Taken from Potatoes Not Prozac, by Kathleen DesMaisons, PhD.

Page | 50

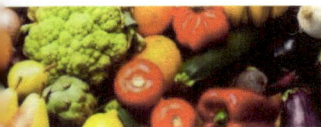

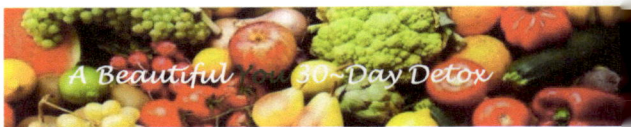

Chapter 11 – Your Transition Diet

**Free Bonus – You may choose a dessert from the
Recipe Section for each day of your Transition**

Day 1

Today is the day you add one grain at breakfast – quinoa. Take note of how you're feeling by adding a grain to your diet. Did it make you feel bloated, sluggish or rundown or are you feeling vigorous, happy or more alive? Don't forget to Journal all of this.

- 7:00 am * Morning Lemon / Lime Regimen
- 8:00 am herbal tea or organic coffee
- 10:00 am Breakfast: SuperFood Quinoa Breakfast Bowl
- 11:30 am Coconut Water (4 ounces) add snack if needed
- 1:30 pm Lunch: Lavish Berry Salad with Fruity Ginger Dressing
- 4:00 pm Snack: 2 tbsp. Raw Hummus (no Beans) with Raw Veggies, Cleansing Flush
- 6:00 pm Dinner: Dijon Corn Salad with Dessert of your liking

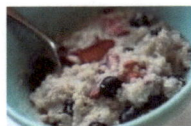

Day 2

No new additions for this day. How are you feeling today, bloated or good? Now that you've eaten quinoa yesterday, write down in your food diary how you're feeling today.

- 7:00 am * Morning Lemon / Lime Regimen
- 8:00 am herbal tea or organic coffee
- 10:00 am Breakfast: Any Smoothie in the Recipe Section that you'd like
- 11:30 am Coconut Water (4 ounces) add snack if needed
- 1:30 pm Lunch: Tomato Fennel Salad
- 4:00 pm Snack: Banana with 2 tbsp. Tahini & unsweetened coconut, Cleansing Flush
- 6:00 pm Dinner: Asparagus Quinoa Risotto, Dessert of your liking

Day 3

Today, you'll be adding a new food – Garbanzo Beans.

- 7:00 am * Morning Lemon / Lime Regimen
- 8:00 am herbal tea or organic coffee
- 10:00 am Breakfast: Chocolate Covered Cherries Smoothie

Page | 51

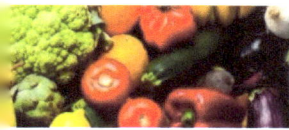

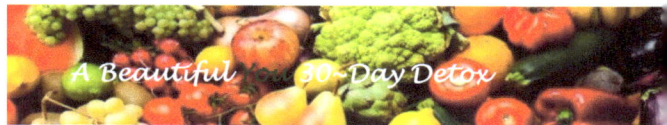

- 11:30 am Coconut Water (4 ounces) add snack if needed
- 1:30 pm Lunch: Mistress of the Citrus Salad
- 4:00 pm Snack: 2 SuperFood Goji Balls, Cleansing Flush
- 6:00 pm Dinner: Moroccan Spiced Bowl, Dessert of your choice

Day 4

YAY! It is your last day of the Transition Diet. Please keep in mind that when you begin to add foods back into your diet from the Elimination List, you risk the chance of developing inflammation again, so please do so with caution. Try to eliminate all processed foods from your diet. If it has a label, then it was manufactured in a plant. Try to stick to foods that are in their natural state.

- 7:00 am * Morning Lemon / Lime Regimen
- 8:00 am herbal tea or organic coffee
- 10:00 am Breakfast: Organic Breakfast Bowl
- 11:30 am Coconut Water (4 ounces) add snack if needed
- 1:30 pm Lunch: Asian Salad, Chopped
- 4:00 pm Snack: 2 tbsp. Italian Hummus (See Recipe) with ½ sweet potato or fresh raw veggies, Cleansing Flush
- 6:00 pm Dinner: Moroccan Quinoa Salad, Dessert of your choice

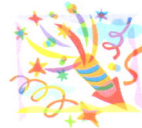

YOU'VE JUST FINISHED YOUR TRANSITION DIET AND DETOX!

Continue eating clean and only add 1 food from the Elimination List at a time to your meals every other day or so. Keep in mind to continue Journaling on how you're feeling emotionally and physically as you make progress. I'm so proud of your...CONGRATS!

Rules for Re-Introducing Foods From the Elimination List Back Into Your Diet

- ✓ Add a food every 2 to 3 days.
- ✓ Eat and cook lightly and simply.
- ✓ Eat regular meals
- ✓ Keep up with your Food Diary, writing it in your Journal every single day.
- ✓ Stay away from foods that you believe are causing you problems or that you might be sensitive to.

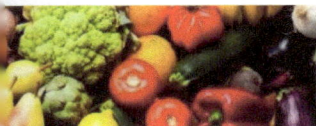

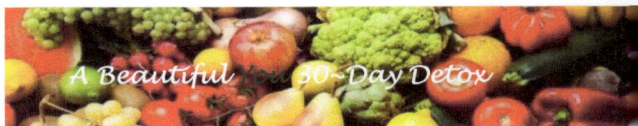

✓ Be your own food police and always read labels if you go that route. (i.e., if you choose to buy hummus instead of making it yourself from scratch, make sure that it's preservative and gluten free). And most of all, if you don't recognize an ingredient in your food, neither can your stomach, liver or kidneys.

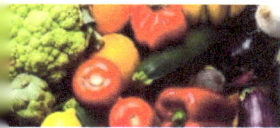

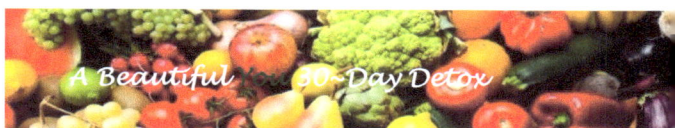

Chapter 12 – Detox I Feel Greats!

Hot Towel Scrubs

Scrubbing your body can be done before or after your bath or shower, or anytime during the day. All you need is a bathroom sink with hot water in it, and a medium – sized cotton (I suggest white) washcloth.

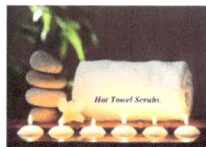

INSTRUCTIONS:

- ❖ Turn on the hot water in your sink and fill it.
- ❖ Hold the towel at both ends and place it in the hot water.
- ❖ Wring out the towel.
- ❖ While the towel is still hot and steamy, begin scrubbing your skin gently.
- ❖ Do only one section at a time: for example, begin with the hands and fingers and work your way up the arms to the shoulders, neck and face, then down to the chest, upper back, abdomen, lower back, buttocks, legs, feet and toes. Make sure to swish the towel several times and wring it out before going on to the next section.
- ❖ Scrub lightly until the skin becomes slightly pink or feels tingly and warm. DO NOT OVER SCRUB!
- ❖ Reheat the towel often by dipping it in the sink of hot water after scrubbing each section, or as soon as the towel begins to cool.

BENEFITS:

- ❖ Reduces muscle aches and tension.
- ❖ Reenergizes in the morning time and deeply relaxes at nighttime.
- ❖ Opens your pours to release toxins
- ❖ Softens deposits of hard fat below your skin and prepares them for discharge.
- ❖ Allows excess fat, mucus, cellulite and toxins to actively discharge to the surface rather than to accumulate around deeper vital organs.
- ❖ Relieves stress through meditative action of rubbing the skin.
- ❖ Activates that lymphatic system, especially when scrubbing underarms and groin.

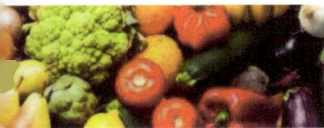

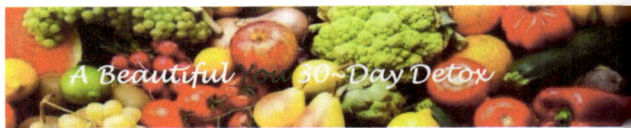

❖ Can be a sacred moment in your day, especially if done with candlelight and a drop or two of essential oil, such as lavender.

❖ Creates a profound and loving relationship with the body, especially parts not often shown: especially helpful for a person with body image problems.

Nourishments for Your Skin

At this particular time or week, you should be using natural soaps and skin/hair products whenever possible to avoid absorbing additional toxic properties into your body.

Your "All Natural" Moisturizer: Coconut Oil.

Coconut Oil can be used as an overnight moisturizer, acne treatment or healing relief from different skin irritations. So, every night before going to bed, apply virgin, organic coconut oil directly onto your face and massage in a circular motion.

Physical Activity

Exercise aids in the release of toxins from your body. It's also important for keeping the blood and lymphatic system flowing. Consistency is key, as it helps relieve stress and toxicity by increasing the blood flow to your brain. Exercise also stimulates the nervous system and releases endorphins into your body. Sweating is also a key component of releasing toxins from your body.

Hydration

HYDRATION is KEY to a successful Detox tool! Focus on flushing out the toxins that invade your body. Your goal is to drink ½ your weight in ounces in water each and every day! OK, let's put it this way…say you weighed 120 pounds, you'll need to drink 60 ounces of water per day. When you drink adequate amounts of water every-day, this will ward off headaches as well as joint pains as your body is releasing toxins. *It's imperative that you don't forgo this step!*

Do Something Rewarding For Yourself Every Day

You can do something as big as a massage or as small as a cup of tea on your porch without your cell phone buzzing in your hand. You can try doing a self-massage or take a bath with a few lavender drops. Also, treat yourself to a good night's sleep by turning out the lights and TV, shut your mind down, put your health and yourself first and just unplug!

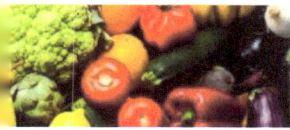

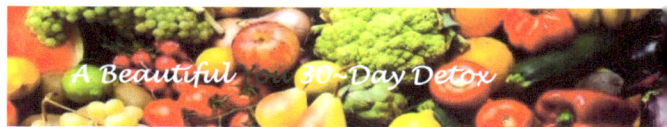

Rewrite Your Inner Narrative

Re-mold the conversations in your head. Energy is most important. Remove all the negativity because it's killing your energy, so don't allow it to creep into your mind or spirit. Now's the perfect time to become aware of what else, other than food, you need to detox from your daily routine.

A Great Epsom Salt Bath

Try taking an Epsom salt bath. Add ½ cup of Epsom salt, ½ cup baking soda and a few drops lavender into a tub of warm water and soak for at least 30 minutes. What Epsom salt does is relax the body, detoxifies the liver and provides your body with the essential mineral, magnesium, which is necessary for optimal relaxation, digestion, detox and health.

Castor Oil Packets

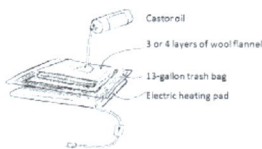

Castor oil
3 or 4 layers of wool flannel
13-gallon trash bag
Electric heating pad

This is an "All Natural" way to rid the organs of toxic build-up.

Making Your Packet:

Take a piece of wool flannel about 12 x 18 inches in size and fold it into 3 thicknesses. You'll need it to be about the same size as the heating pad that you'll be using so that the pad heats the entire packet but does not touch your skin. Put the wool in a pan, such as a large disposable baking pan, and pour enough castor oil over it. Let this sit until the wool is well saturated. Notice how after each use, you'll probably need to add a little castor oil. You'll be able to reuse the packet many, many times. When you're not using it, store it in a plastic baggie in the refrigerator.

Packet Placement:

You should be lying down with your packet on the right side of your body, extended from a little bit above the bottom of your breastbone or sternum, to about 4 inches below your navel. The packet should wrap around the body on your right side, from the navel as far as the side as you can get it.

Guidelines for using your packet:

Use your packet in the evening right before bedtime. Spread out a large plastic garbage bag on the bed so that the oil won't leak onto your bed. Fold a towel, make sure it's an old towel, because the oil is just about impossible to wash out completely, and place on the

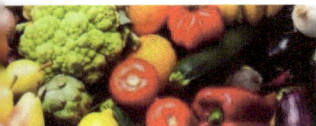

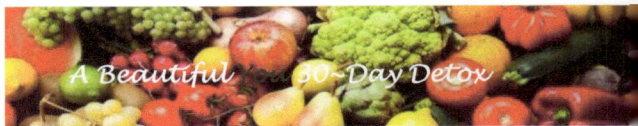

garbage bag. Take the cloth cover off of the heating pad and place the heating pad on top of the towel. It's important to heat the packet before you put it onto your body. You can either heat it in the oven on a low temp setting for about 15 minutes or heat it in a microwave oven in a microwave safe container, for about one minute or so, or you can simply turn on the heating pad and set it on high, put the packet onto the heating pad and let it get warm for a few minutes before putting it onto your body. BE CAREFUL! If you're not sure of what's too hot or high, start with a slightly warm session and work up to a warmer one. If it's not warm enough at this phase, it may help to rest your arms and hands on the towel to press the packet more firmly against your body.

Lay on your back on the plastic bag. Put the packet on your abdomen with the heating pad on top and towel on top of that. Make sure that the heating pad control is easily accessible of your hand as you may need to adjust it so that the packet does not become too hot or cold.

Keep the packet on for 1 to 1 ½ hours, and have a paper towel on hand to wipe off the oil when you're done and ready to get up, and again, make sure that you don't get any into your bed. If need be, combine baking soda with warm water, (2 tsp. per quart) and use the solution with paper towels or a sponge to clean off the castor oil. You may also want to take a shower with soap after your packet.

Best when used for 3 days in a row and take 4 days off, then repeat again.

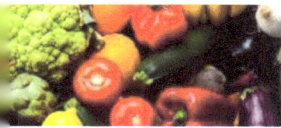

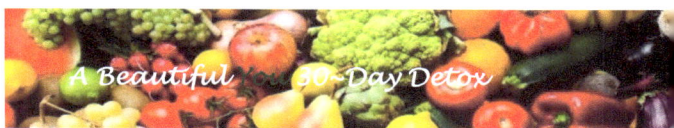

Chapter 13 – Your Detox Meal Recipes

Fantabulous Smoothies!

For the smoothie recipes, just add all ingredients, (except greens for green smoothies) into a VitaMix or high-speed blender. When adding greens, first break up fruit in blender, then add greens. Add water when needed to reach the desired consistency. If possible, use organic fruits and vegetables. You can add extra protein to any smoothie by adding 3 tbsp. hemp seeds. Most recipes in this section, unless otherwise noted, is one serving.

Thin Mint Fat Busting Smoothie

1 cup coconut, rice or hemp milk
¾ coconut water
1 tbsp. ground flax or chia seed
½ avocado
1 tsp. peppermint extract
½ cup ice (optional)

Black & Strawberry Dreamcicle Smoothie

1 cup coconut, rice or hemp milk
1 cup frozen blackberries
½ cup strawberries
½ avocado
½ tsp. vanilla
1 – 2 tbsp. ground flax or chia seed
Ice (optional)

Creaminess with a lil' Kick

1 cup coconut water, coconut, rice or hemp milk
½ bunch kale
1 banana
½ orange
1 tsp. vanilla
1 tsp cinnamon
1 dash cayenne
1 – 2 tbsp. ground flax or chia seed
½ cup ice (optional)

Chocolate Covered Cherries

4 – 6 ounces coconut water
1 banana
1 cup frozen cherries
½ cup mango
1 handful collard greens (I promise you'll never taste them)
1 tbsp. raw cacao nibs ground
1 – 2 tbsp. flax or chia seed

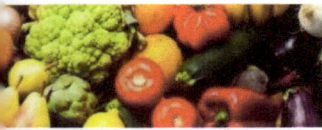

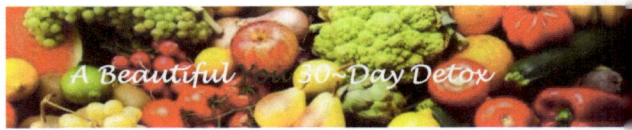

Greased Lightning Smoothie

1 banana
1 orange
1 cup coconut water
1 cup filtered water
2 tbsp. pumpkin seeds
1 tbsp. ground flax seed
1 tbsp. hemp seeds
1 tbsp. raw honey, agave or 5 drops stevia
1 tbsp. coconut oil

Sassy RAW Smoothie

1 banana
1 cup coconut water, hemp or rice milk
1 tbsp. ground flax seed
1 handful spinach or kale
1 cup frozen berries
1 splash vanilla extract
Ice (optional)

Thunderbolt with a Dash of Sunshine

2 organic kiwis, peeled & chopped
1 large mango
2 cups fresh spinach
1 cup coconut water
1 cup hemp or rice milk
Ice (optional)

Sleek & Sassy Smoothie

¾ cup unsweetened coconut, hemp or rice milk
½ cup frozen mixed berries
½ avocado
1 tsp. ground flax seed
1 tsp ground chia seed
1 handful spinach

Summer of Love Smoothie

½ small watermelon, diced
½ banana
2 sticks fennel
1 handful fresh spearmint
½ cup coconut water
Handful of ice (enjoy this smoothie over ice or blend 1 cup of ice into it to make it slushier)

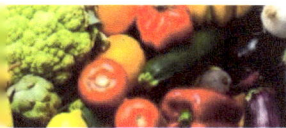

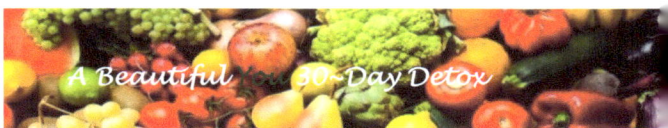

Pear of Lovers Green Smoothie

2 pears, chopped
1 cucumber, chopped
¼ avocado
1 cup spinach
Juice of 1 lime
½ inch piece of ginger
½ cup filtered water, coconut water or coconut milk
Ice (optional)
Stevia or raw honey (optional)

Pineapple Orange Delight Smoothie

1 large orange, peeled & deseeded
1 cup fresh pineapple, cubed
2 cups organic baby spinach, chopped
2 organic stalks celery
½ to 1/3 filtered water
1 tbsp. flax or chia seed ground
2 – 3 cups ice (optional)

Banana – Mango Tropics Smoothie

1 banana
½ - 1 mango
1 tbsp. flax or chia seed, ground
4 – 6 ounces of coconut or filtered water

Orange – Cantaloupe Hit the Tropics Smoothie

1 large orange, peeled & deseeded
1 cup cubed cantaloupe
1 tbsp. flax or chia seed ground
A little coconut or filtered water if needed

Banilla – Orange Smoothie

1 large banana
1 -2 inches chopped vanilla bean
1 large orange, peeled and deseed
1 tbsp. flax or chia seed, ground
4 – 6 ounces coconut or filtered water

Carrot – Apricot Delight Smoothie

2 apricots
1 apple
2 cups fresh baby spinach
2 whole carrots
1 – 2 tbsp. flax or chia seed, ground
½ coconut or filtered water

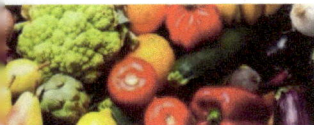

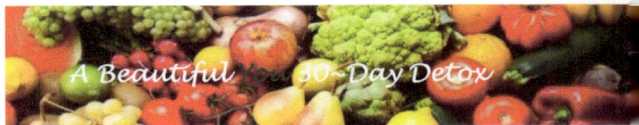

Fruity Zucchini Smoothie

1 medium zucchini
½ cup organic fresh parsley, chopped
2 stalks celery, organic
1 cup pineapple, diced
1 – 2 tbsp. flax or chia seed, ground
4 – 6 ounces coconut or filtered water

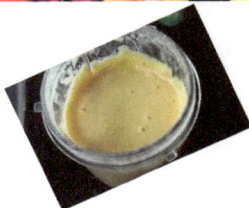

Banananza Smoothie

1 banana
1 large organic apple
1 organic zucchini, chopped
1 tbsp. flax or chia seed, ground
4 – 6 ounces coconut or filtered water

Smoothie with a Kick

2 large, organic carrots, chopped
¼ avocado
1 whole organic apple, cored
2 handfuls baby fresh, organic baby spinach
1 tbsp. fresh grated ginger root
1 tbsp. flax or chia seed, ground
4 – 6 ounces coconut or filtered water

Apple Delight

1 organic apple, cored
½ avocado
1 – 2 tbsp. hemp
2 cups fresh organic spinach
½ - ¾ cup coconut or filtered water
Few ice cubes to make it colder

Happy Cucumber "N" Melon Smoothie

1 organic cucumber, unpeeled
2 cups or ½ ripe honeydew melon
1 tsp. lemon juice
1 ½ tbsp. flax or chia seed, ground
2 tbsp. chopped fresh mint (I prefer Spearmint)
½ cup coconut or filtered water

Cantaloupe Delight Smoothie

1 cucumber, unpeeled
2 cups or ½ ripe cantaloupe, diced
1 tsp. lime juice

Page | 61

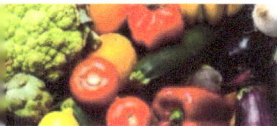

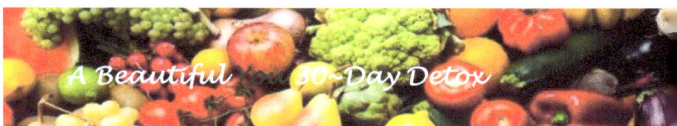

1 tbsp. hemp
2 cups baby spinach
½ cup coconut or filtered water

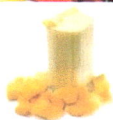

Simply Nourishing Smoothie

1 medium, organic cucumber, unpeeled
1 cup papaya, cubed
½ avocado peeled & pitted
1 tbsp. flax or chia seed
½ cup coconut or filtered water

Great Day-In-The-Morning Smoothie

Meat & 4 – 6 ounces of water from one coconut
1 organic, Fuji apple, cored
¼ avocado
1 tbsp. hemp
2 handfuls fresh organic baby spinach

Peachy – Keen Smoothie

½ - 1 cup coconut water
Meat from 1 young coconut
1 organic peach
½ banana
1 tbsp. flax or chia seed
 2 cups fresh, organic baby spinach

Papapple Smoothie

2 ½ cups cubed papaya
1 organic apple, cored
1 tbsp. flax or chia seed
2 cups organic baby spinach
½ - 1 cup coconut or filtered water

Banana – Strawberry Smoothie

1 banana, peeled
1 cup whole organic strawberries
1 tbsp. hemp
2 cups organic baby spinach
1 medium carrot, chopped
½ - 1 cup coconut or filtered water

Mango Tango Smoothie

1 cup pineapple, cubed
1 large mango peeled and pitted
1 tbsp. hemp

Page | 62

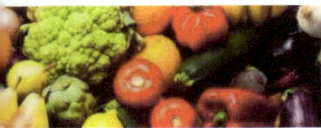

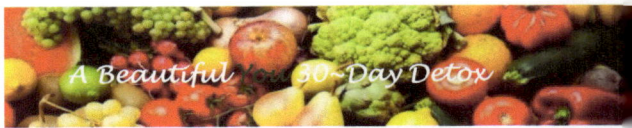

2 cups baby spinach
½ - 1 cup coconut or filtered water

Orange Madness Smoothie

2 ½ cups papaya
1 orange, peeled
1 pear, cored
1 organic celery stalk
1 tbsp. flax or chia seed
2 cups fresh, organic baby spinach
½ - 1 cup coconut or filtered water

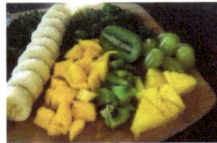

Vanilla – Pineapple Sunrise Smoothie

1 cup pineapple, cubed
1 banana, peeled
1 vanilla bean
1 ½ tbsp. hemp
2 cups organic baby spinach, fresh of course
1 organic celery stalk
4 – 6 ounces coconut or filtered water

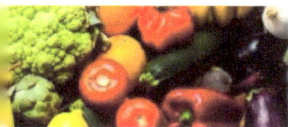

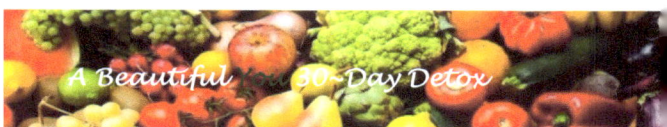

Juicing
Liquid Gold!

For all of the juice recipes, juice each ingredient together in your VitaMix or Juicer. To sweeten any Juice, just add vanilla extract, stevia in the raw, raw honey or juice from a lemon or lime. If you like it with a little kick, you may add hot sauce or cayenne pepper, cinnamon or nutmeg. Keep in mind to use organic whenever possible. Also remember to wash your produce thoroughly if you wish to include the rind or peel in your juice.

When or if you're using your blender, make sure to consult the manufacturer's instructions for juicing.

Hydration Station

2 – 3 cucumbers
2 green apples
¼ beet or handful of organic strawberries
Fresh mint to taste (Optional
~Serves 2

Luscious Skin Green Goodness

2 green apples
2 cucumbers
2 handfuls fresh spinach
2 large carrots
4 stalks celery
1 lemon peeled and deseeded
~ add 1 cup coconut water after you've juiced all ingredients together
~ Serves 2

Let's Go Wild

½ papaya
½ pineapple
1 cucumber, unpeeled
3 handfuls fresh organic spinach or kale
Juice of 1 lemon and juice of 1 lime
3 drops of vanilla extract (optional)

Not your Momma's Green Juice

3 celery stalks
1 cucumber with skin
2 handfuls romaine lettuce
2 handfuls baby spinach
2 pears
1 handful parsley

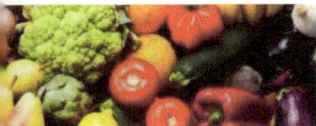

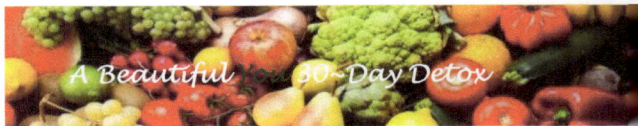

1 handful cilantro
4 ounces coconut water
Vanilla extract or stevia (optional)
~ add 1 cup coconut water after you've juiced all ingredients

Goodness Gracious Green Juice

4 celery stalks
½ green apple
1 cucumber, sliced lengthwise
3 kale leaves
1 lemon, juiced

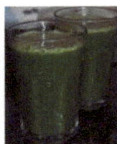

Mean Green Mojito

3 kale leaves
½ cup spinach
4 celery stalks
1 cucumber, sliced lengthwise
1 lemon, juiced
1 lime, juiced
½ green apple
3 sprigs mint
Ginger (optional)
Stevia, agave or honey to sweeten

The Anti-Wrinkle Green Juice

2 tomatoes
1 cucumber with skin
2 celery stalks
1 garlic clove
Pinch sea salt
1 lime, peeled

Cucumber – Grapefruit Juice

1 green apple, chopped
2 celery ribs
1 cucumber, sliced lengthwise
1 grapefruit, peeled and deseeded
1 cup kale

Flowing Digestion Juice

1 pinch ginger
1 cup diced pineapple
1 chopped green apple
3 mint sprigs
2 ounces Aloe Vera juice (optional)

Page | 65

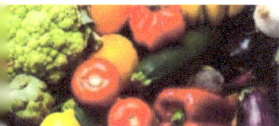

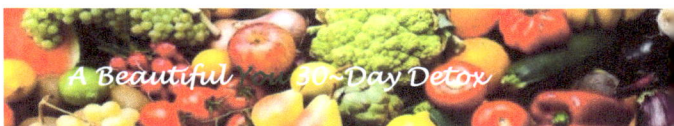

Oh My Healthy Liver

1 cucumber
½ lemon with rind
6 asparagus spears, washed thoroughly

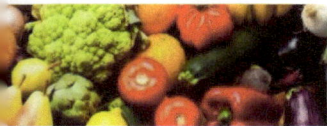

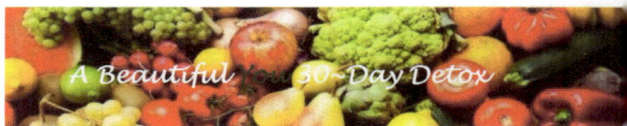

DIPS

For this section, if you can't find nutritional yeast, simply omit it from the recipe. If you're intolerant to soy and/or miso, just remove it from the recipe as well.

Tahini Dip

½ cup tahini (sesame paste)
1 clove garlic, minced
1 lemon, juiced
¼ cup water
1 – 2 tbsp. Wheat Free Tamari (optional)

Whisk or blend all the ingredients until creamy. Slowly add more water to get the desired consistency. This dip will thicken in the fridge and can be stored for upwards to 3 days.

Raw Bean Free Hummus

2 organic zucchini chopped
¾ cup raw tahini
½ cup fresh lemon juice
1 tbsp. nutritional yeast
3 cloves garlic

Blend all the ingredients in a VitaMix or high speed blender and enjoy!

Mexicali Dip

½ red bell pepper, chopped
1 yellow squash, chopped
2 tbsp. tahini
Juice of 1 lemon
1/8 tsp cayenne
1/8 tsp salt
2 tbsp. nutritional yeast

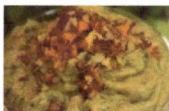

Blend all ingredients in high speed blender. Served with a croup-d-tae (raw veggies), cooked veggies, in a lettuce wrap with avocado, or eat alone as a raw soup.

Detoxing Pesto

1 cup cleaned, loosely packed fresh basil leaves
½ cup fresh sorrel leaves, cilantro or mint
2 sundried tomatoes
2 cloves freshly peeled garlic
Juice of 1 lemon
¼ - ½ cup good quality, cold pressed extra virgin olive oil, as needed
Grey sea salt, to taste

Page | 67

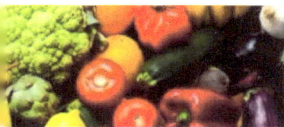

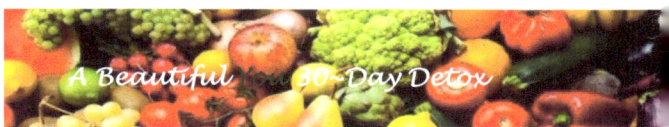

Combine the basil, sorrel, sun-dried tomatoes, lemon juice and garlic in a food processor bowl; pulse and process the mixture until finely chopped. Slowly add EVOO in a steady drizzle as you pulse the processor on and off. Process until it becomes a smooth, light paste. Add enough EVOO to keep your pesto moist and spreadable. Season with grey sea salt. Cover tightly and chill in the fridge for at least 1 hour to marry the flavors. If storing overnight, pour a thin layer of EVOO over the top of the pesto to help keep it bright green.

Peach Salsa

2 tomatoes
2 peaches
1 clove finely minced garlic
1 jalapeno, finely minced (remove seeds for less heat)
1 lime, juiced
1 tbsp. fresh cilantro
1 finely minced shallot
Grey sea salt to taste

Chop peaches and tomatoes and add garlic and shallots. Toss in jalapeno, lime juice and cilantro. Sprinkle grey sea salt if needed. Use this salsa in lettuce wraps or in celery sticks

Sweet Potato – Sage Dip

2 chopped sweet potatoes
½ avocado
1 tbsp. coconut oil
1 clove garlic
½ tsp. cinnamon
2 sage leaves or ¼ tsp. dried sage
¼ tsp grey sea salt

Cook sweet potatoes in small pot with enough water to cover. Boil until potatoes are tender, bout 10 minutes. Drain excess water and add to food processer and process. Add remaining ingredients and blend until smooth.

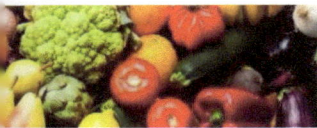

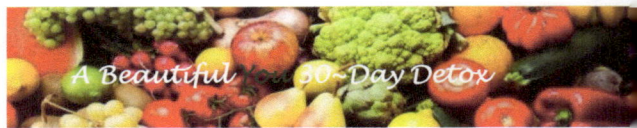

RAW MEALS

Detox Your Body Lettuce Wraps

6 lettuce leaves
1 avocado
¼ cup sauerkraut or kimchee
1 diced tomato
1 tbsp. hemp seed
1 cup sprouts of your choice
1 – 2 tbsp. tahini dressing

Lay out the lettuce leaves and place all ingredients onto each leaf and roll up. Add 1 – 2 tbsp. tahini dressing for extra flavoring or a dash of cayenne pepper for a little kick. *Serves 2*

Tomato – Fennel Salad

2 cups chopped butter leaf lettuce
1 cup chopped cherry tomatoes
¼ cup chopped fennel
1 tbsp. fresh mint
1 tbsp. pumpkin seeds
1 – 2 tbsp. tahini dressing

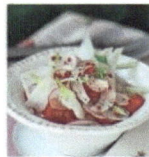

Make the tahini dressing per recipe. In a large bowl, put your lettuce first then add chopped tomatoes, fennel, mint, pumpkin seeds and then top with tahini dressing. *Serves 2*

Beach Body Slaw

6 – 7 cups of roughly chopped red/purple cabbage
1 carrot peeled and shaved into strips
3 chopped celery stalks
1 red bell pepper, sliced thinly
2 handfuls freshly chopped parsley
4 tbsp. black sesame seeds
Salt & pepper to taste
1 – 2 tahini dressing

In a large bowl, combine the chopped celery, pepper, cabbage, shaved carrot and parsley. Add black sesame seeds and drizzle with tahini dressing for a creamy consistency. *Serves 4*

Mistress of the Citrus Salad

1 bunch of romaine lettuce, torn into bite-size pieces
2 grapefruits, peeled and deseeded, chopped
1 lemon juiced
¼ red onion, finely chopped
2 tbsp. minced fresh parsley
1/8 cup toasted pumpkin seeds
Grey sea salt and pepper to taste

Page | 69

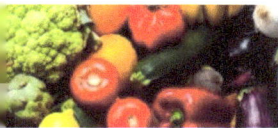

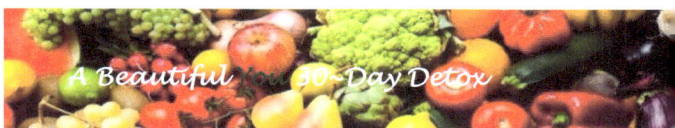

Place romaine in large bowl and top with grapefruit, red onion and parsley. Squeeze on lemon juice and sprinkle with pumpkin seeds, salt and pepper. *Serves 4*

Orange ~ Arugula Salad

1 cup arugula
2 cups spinach
2 oranges, peeled and sliced
½ cup cherry tomatoes halved
2 tbsp. pine nuts
1 avocado, diced
1 – 2 tbsp. simple miso dressing, tahini dressing or juice of 1 lime

Place salad greens in large bowl. Place cherry tomatoes, oranges, avocado and pine nuts on top. Toss in dressing before serving. *Serves 2*

Sweet & Sexy Detox Salad

2 cups spinach
1 lemon, juiced
1 apple, small diced
1/8 cup pumpkin seeds
¼ cup fresh berries of your liking
2 tbsp. parsley
¼ small diced red onion
Drizzle of tahini dressing
Grey sea salt and pepper to taste

In large bowl, add spinach, half of lemon juice and a drizzle of tahini dressing and a little sea salt. Massage until spinach begins to wilt for about 2 minutes. Top with apples, pumpkin seeds, berries, onions and parsley. *Serves 2*

Dijon Corn Salad

By: Rachel Feldman
2 cups arugula, spinach, frisee, or other leafy greens of your choice
2 cups fresh raw corn
½ cup cherry tomatoes, chopped
2 tsp. Dijon mustard
1 tsp. honey
½ lemon, juiced
Grey sea salt and pepper to taste
EVOO or water (optional)

Combine Dijon mustard, honey and lemon juice in a small mixing bowl. Add olive oil or water to thin to desired consistency. In large bowl, lay out the greens of your choice with fresh corn and tomatoes. Pour dressing on top. Salt and pepper to taste. *Serves 2*

Delicious Asian Salad

1 cup kale, rolled in a cylindrical fashion and sliced thin
1 cup spinach

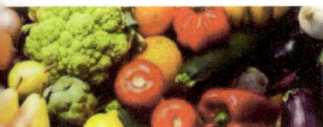

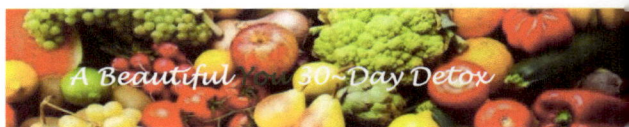

1 cup chopped carrots
1 cup sprouts
1 cup chopped snap peas
3 scallions thinly sliced on a diagonal
1 avocado, ½ for salad and ½ for dressing
2 tbsp. sunflower seed butter or tahini
½ tsp garlic powder
1 lime, juiced
1 tbsp. Bragg's Apple Cider Vinegar
1 tsp. raw honey
¼ cup water.

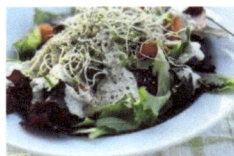

Put the kale in a large mixing bowl and massage until it becomes wilted and tender for about 2 minutes. Add greens, avocado, carrots, snap peas, sprouts and scallions to bowl with kale. To make the dressing, combine ½ of the avocado, 2 tbsp. sunflower butter or tahini, garlic, lime juice, vinegar, honey and water. Toss the salad ingredients in this dressing before serving. *Serves 2*

Warm Spinach Salad

6 cups spinach
2 tsp. EVOO
1 lemon, juiced
1 chopped tomato
1 tsp. grey sea salt
2 tbsp. nutritional yeast (optional)
Your spinach gets this warm texture when massaged. Use your hands to wilt the spinach by combing the spinach in a bowl with grey sea salt and massage until it turns limp. Add EVOO, lemon and yeast. Add tomato on top. *Serves 2*

Minty Watermelon Salad

2 cups mixed greens
1 cup small cubed watermelon
1 tbsp. finely minced mint
1 lime, juiced
½ jalapeno pepper, deseeded and finely minced

Put watermelon into a large bowl. Add mint and jalapeno to melon squeeze fresh lime juice over top and stir to combine. Place on top of mixed greens and enjoy! *Serves 2*

Lavish Berry Salad with Ginger Pineapple Dressing

4 cups spinach
1 cup sprouts of your choice
1 cup chopped strawberries
1 cup blueberries
1 – 2 tbsp. ginger – pineapple dressing

Put strawberries in a bowl with spinach and blueberries and top with sprouts and dressing. *Serves 2*

Page | 71

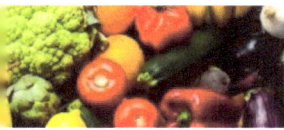

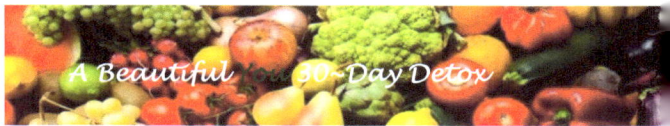

Fruity Zucchini Salad

2 zucchini, spiraled
½ cup chopped strawberries
½ cup chopped asparagus
2 tbsp. pumpkin seeds
½ cup Detoxing Pesto
Grey sea salt and pepper to taste

Spiraled zucchini using a spiralizer or veggie peeler into noodle shape. Do not use the seeds. Add strawberries and asparagus to the bowl of noodles. Add seeds and pesto and combine. *Serves 2*

Mediterranean Kale Salad

4 de-stemmed kale leaves
1 tsp. EVOO
1 ½ tsp. fresh lemon juice
1/8 tsp. grey sea salt
¼ of a red pepper, diced
1 tbsp. pine nuts
1 tbsp. black sliced black olives
Black pepper to taste

Stack kale leaves and roll into a cylindrical shape, like a cigar. Cut into thin strips and then change positions and chop kale into smaller pieces a few times. Put into a medium bowl along with olive oil, lemon juice and salt. Massage kale until it wilts and looks cooked. Add remaining ingredients and toss gently. Add pepper to taste. *Serves 2 – 4*

Cress Salad with Golden Beets

1 peeled and sliced golden beet
½ cup cress
3 scallions
1 lime, juiced and zest
1 tbsp. Dijon mustard
2 tbsp. EVOO
Grey sea salt to taste

Toss beets, scallions and cress together in bowl. Add lime juice, zest, Dijon and EVOO. Toss to coat. Add grey sea salt and pepper to taste. *Serves 2*

Raw Pasta with Marinara

2 peeled zucchini
1 Roma tomato, ripe
½ cup chopped sundried tomatoes, bout ½ cup soaked or in oil. I prefer in oil.
½ chopped red pepper, bout ½ cup
2 tbsp. EVOO
3 tsp. fresh oregano
1 tbsp. fresh basil
½ tsp. grated or crushed garlic
¼ plus 1/8 tsp. grey sea salt

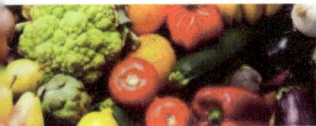

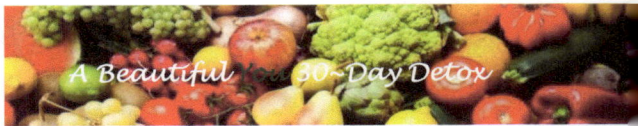

Black & Cayenne pepper for a little kick

Spiral zucchini and set aside in a mesh strainer to drain the water that may build up. Add all ingredients into a small food processor. Stop the food processor every now and then to scrape down the sides. Process to desired texture, smooth or chunky. *Serves 2*

Jicama Salad with Smashing Curry Sauce

1 large jicama, cubed
1 cup chopped pea pods
2 chopped scallions
½ cup raisins or currants
½ smashing curry sauce

Peel and cut jicama into ¼" pieces. Cut pea pods into 1/3 pieces. Combine jicama, pea pods, raisins or currants and scallions. Add ½ of the smashing curry sauce

Smashing Curry Sauce

1/3 to ½ cup tahini
Flesh from 1 young coconut
¼ coconut water
2 tsp. curry powder
1 tsp. grey sea salt

Open coconut and drain water out. Keep water. Remove flesh and place ¼ coconut water into a blender. Add flesh of coconut, 1/3 to ½ cup tahini, curry powder and sea salt. Combine until smooth.

Luscious Summer Salad

To prepare this recipe, do it a day in advance because you have to dehydrate the ingredients to create the brittle.
DRESSING:
8 medium strawberries
1 cup EVOO
¼ cup maple syrup
2 lemons juiced
Place all ingredients into blender and blend until smooth.

BRITTLE:

1 cup pumpkin seeds
1 ½ tbsp. cinnamon
1 ½ tbsp. ginger
Pinch cayenne pepper

Place all ingredients except the pumpkin seeds in a food processor and pulse until well ground. Add seeds and pulse, making sure some of the seeds remain in small chunks. If you need a little more moisture, add just a touch of maple syrup. But it shouldn't be too loose as you're trying to make a brittle. Flatten out onto a teflex sheet for a food dehydrator and dehydrate for at least 8 hours or until brittle is very dry. If you don't have a dehydrator, place in oven on a non-stick baking sheet, continuously checking for doneness.

Page | 73

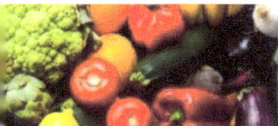

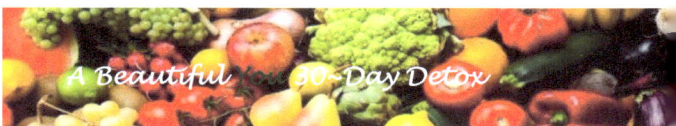

THE SALAD

4 cups of greens of our choice
Strawberry vinaigrette
16 strawberries

To assemble, place salad greens in center of plate. Surround with halved strawberries. Drizzle with strawberry vinaigrette and top with pumpkin seed brittle. *Serves 2 – 4*

Peachy Kale Salad with Miso Vinaigrette

1 large bunch kale
2 peaches, peeled and cubed
1 coarsely chopped cup of pecans

VINAIGRETTE:

2 tbsp. grade b maple syrup
2 tbsp. EVOO
1 tbsp. Bragg's Apple Cider Vinegar
2 tsp. light miso
Grey sea salt and pepper to taste

Remove kale from stems and tear into bite-sized pieces. Put in a large bowl. Prepare vinaigrette in a small bowl. Pour vinaigrette over kale and massage the dressing into the leaves, wilting them. Remember, this is a vital step. Throw in peaches and pecans. *Serves 2 – 4*

Berry ~ Mango Salad

1 head romaine lettuce
1 cup sliced strawberries
1 cup diced mango
1 cup small diced jicama
1 diced avocado
1 cup pumpkin seeds or pine nuts

BLUEBERRY VINAIGRETTE:

1 cup blueberries
1 tbsp. maple syrup
2 tbsp. red wine vinegar
¼ cup EVOO

Blend and combine vinaigrette ingredients to consistency that suites you. Refrigerate to marry flavors. Rip romaine and place onto a plate. Mix fruit and jicama. Put a handful of fruit mixture on top lettuce bed. Add vinaigrette. *Serves 4 - 6*

Luscious Melon Salad with Mint

6 cups 1" cubed watermelon or melon of your choice
2 cups ¼" cubed jicama
¾ cup red onion

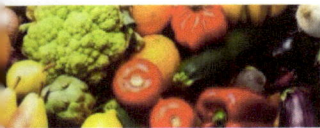

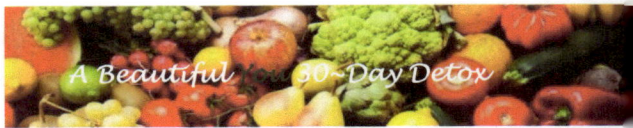

2 tbsp. fresh chopped mint
Grey sea salt and pepper to taste

Combine all ingredients and let stand in the fridge for a while to marry flavors before serving. *Serves 4 – 6*

Heirloom Tomatoes with a Mexi ~ Cali Salad

3 cups heirloom tomatoes, cubed if larger and halved is smaller
2 cubed avocados
4 ears fresh corn removed from its cob
½ very thinly sliced purple onion

Mix all ingredients then pour dressing over veggies and toss gently

MEXI ~ CALI DRESSING:

½ cup soaked cashews. Soak for at least 6 hours
½ cup water
1 tbsp. EVOO
2 tbsp. fresh lime juice
¼ tsp. ground chipotle
¼ tsp. smoked paprika
Grey sea salt and pepper to taste

Combine all dressing ingredients in a blender and blend until smooth. *Serves 4 – 6*

Dressed Up Zucchini with Veggies

MARINADE:

2 tbsp. lemon juice
1 tbsp. maple syrup
1 tsp. fresh grated ginger
1/3 cup EVOO
1 tsp. thyme

Mix all ingredients together.

MUSHROOMS:

2 Portobello mushrooms
¼ cup EVOO
3 tbsp. tamari
2 tbsp. maple syrup

Cut mushrooms into slices. Mix together EVOO, tamari and maple syrup. Pour this mixture over the mushrooms and marinate over night. To assemble:

2 spiraled zucchini
2 grated carrots
2 scallions
Marinated mushrooms
½ cup pumpkin seeds

Page | 75

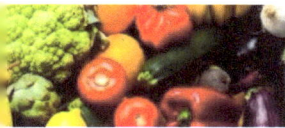

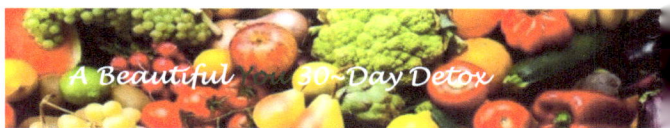

Place zucchini noodles in bowl, pour marinade over and let stand in fridge overnight. Drain noodles and place in a circle onto the plate. Mix together carrots, scallions, mushrooms and pumpkin seeds. Put in the middle of noodle nest. *Serves 4 – 6*

Maple Dancing on the Tongue Slaw

SLAW:

2 apples
½ lemon
2 cups small diced butternut squash
2 lbs. broccoli stems, shredded
2 stalks celery
1 cup dried cranberries
¾ cup pumpkin seeds

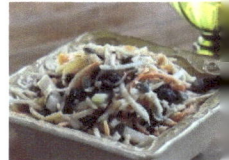

Put apples in bowl and squeeze juice from lemon and stir. Add the rest of the ingredients.

MAPLE DRESSING:

¾ cup tahini
½ cup water
1 lemon, juiced
2 tsp. freshly grated ginger
3 tbsp. maple syrup
Pinch grey sea salt

Wisk together and pour over slaw. *Serves 2 – 4*

Carrot Curry Salad

4 cups grated carrots, (10 Medium carrots)
2 cups snow peas
2 cups fresh pineapple
½ cup raisins or currants
1 thinly sliced, bunch of scallions

CURRY DRESSING:

½ cups cashews, soaked for at least 6 hours and drained
½ cup almond milk
2 tsp. sweet yellow curry powder
½ tsp. tamari
1 tbsp. maple syrup
Grey sea salt to taste

Toss carrots, snow peas, pineapple, raisins or currants and scallions together in a large bowl. Put all dressing ingredients in a high-speed blender and blend until smooth. Pour over salad and mix through to coat. *Serves 6*

Marinated Cucumbers

2 very thinly sliced cucumbers

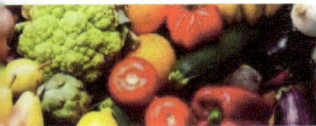

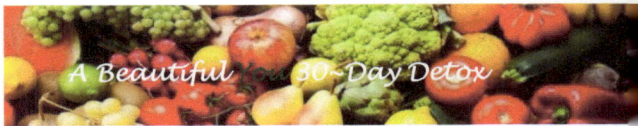

1 very thinly sliced sweet onion

MARINADE:

½ cup Bragg's apple cider vinegar
½ cup water
½ lemon, juiced
2 tbsp. maple syrup
Grey sea salt and pepper
1 tsp. chili flakes

Mix marinade ingredients together. Toss in cucumbers and onions and let marinade overnight. Serves 2 – 4

The Radish Has it Salad with Curry Vinaigrette

SALAD:

1 head butter lettuce
10 radishes
1 mandarin orange, segmented
¼ cup pecans, soaked and dehydrated
½ cup cilantro, leaves only
1 pomegranate, seeded (if in season) if not, try dried

Combine all ingredients in a bowl and set aside.

DRESSING:

1 tsp madras curry powder mix
2 tbsp. lemon juice
½ cup EVOO
2 tbsp. white miso
¼ cup orange juice
1 grated shallot
1 tsp. honey
½ tsp. grey sea salt

Blend all ingredients in a high speed blender. Add to salad when ready to serve. *Serves 2 – 4*

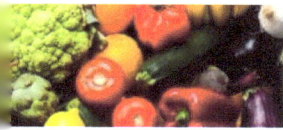

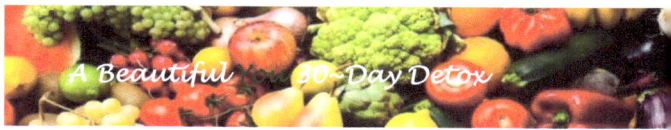

COOKED MEALS

IF YOU DON'T HAVE A STEAMER, JUST BOIL YOUR VEGGIES WITH A LITTLE
FILTERED WATER UNTIL TENDER, BUT STILL HAS A BITE TO THEM.

Healthy Bowl with Orange Zest

1 small head of broccoflower, chopped into bite-sized pieces
1 small head of cauliflower, chopped into bite-sized pieces
Zest of 1 orange
2 tbsp. EVOO
¼ cup hemp or pumpkin seeds
Grey sea salt and pepper

Steam broccoflower and cauliflower until tender. Drain and toss with EVOO, zest and grey
sea salt and pepper and top with seeds. *Serves 2*

Curried Butternut Squash with Broccoli

1 good sized butternut squash, peeled and diced
1 head broccoli, chopped
2 tbsp. coconut oil
¼ tsp curry powder
¼ tsp. garlic powder
Dash of cinnamon
1 tbsp. fresh cilantro
Grey sea salt and pepper to taste

Steam squash and broccoli until tender. Steam squash first for 10 minutes then add broccoli
for the last 5 minutes. Drain both then mash the squash with coconut oil and spices. Toss
the broccoli in at the end and top with cilantro. *Serves 2*

Coconut Brussels Sprouts with Golden Beets

2 cups chopped Brussels Sprouts
2 large chopped golden beets
2 tbsp. coconut oil
2 tbsp. dried coconut flakes
½ tsp. garlic powder
Grey sea salt and pepper to taste

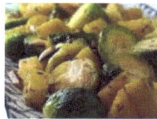

Steam Brussels sprouts and beets until tender, bout 10 minutes. Drain, add to a bowl, and
top with coconut oil, coconut flakes, garlic, salt and pepper. Stir to combine. Sprinkle with
extra coconut flakes to garnish. *Serves 2*

Spicy Tex ~ Mex Wrap

4 collard leaves, de-stemmed
½ cup adzuki beans
1 cup chopped tomato
1 avocado, chopped
Juice of 1 lime
¼ tsp. coriander

Page | 78

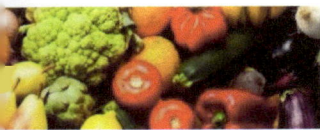

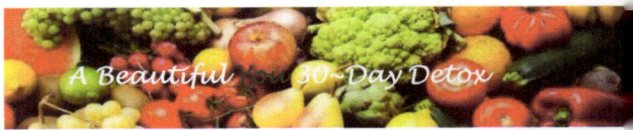

1/8 tsp cayenne
1/8 tsp chipotle powder
1 tsp cumin
Peach Salsa or Mexicali Dip

Combine adzuki beans, tomato and avocado in a bowl and toss in lime juice and spices. Use collard greens as a wrap for the mixture. Add Salsa or Dip if desired. *Serves 2*

Confetti Rice

2 cups cauliflower, chopped
1 red bell pepper, chopped
3 carrots, chopped
½ mango, chopped
3 scallion, thinly sliced
¼ red onion, chopped
1 tbsp. sesame seeds
1 tsp. sesame oil
Grey sea salt and pepper to taste

Steam cauliflower until tender or about 10 minutes. Drain and process in a food processor until it's a rice-like consistency. Add all other ingredients and toss. *Serves 2*

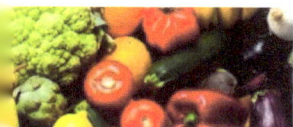

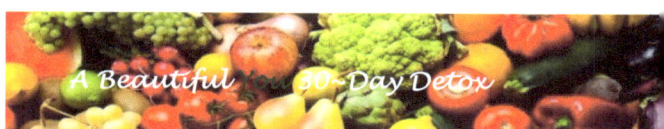

RAW SOUPS

Yummy Raw Tomato Bisque

3 chopped tomatoes
10 sundried tomatoes
1 zucchini
2 tbsp. tahini
½ avocado
½ cup hot water
2 garlic cloves
1 tbsp. fresh basil
½ tbsp. fresh thyme
½ tbsp. fresh oregano
1 jalapeno, for a little kick

Blend all the ingredients in a blender until smooth and warm, say bout 3 minutes. You can top with fresh sprouts, halved cherry tomatoes or slices of avocado. *Serves 2*

Love Your Skin Soup

1 chopped tomato
1 chopped small yam
2 peeled and chopped carrot
1 small yellow squash, chopped
5 sun-dried tomatoes
Pinch of cayenne
Pinch of cumin
¼ tsp. turmeric
¼ tsp. curry powder
Fresh basil, optional
1 tsp. white miso past or ¼ tsp. grey sea salt
1 small chopped zucchini

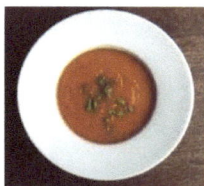

Blend all ingredients until smooth. Top with halved cherry tomato, sliced avocado or with a dollop of coconut cream. *Serves 2*

Not Yo Momma's Chicken Soup (Vegan)

1 cup filtered water, plus more if needed
1 cup chopped celery
1 cup cauliflower
1 cup chopped yellow squash
2 tbsp. fresh dill, minced
2 cloves garlic, minced
1 tbsp. white miso paste
Grey sea salt and pepper to taste
1 zucchini, spiraled
¼ avocado, diced

Steam cauliflower until tender, say 10 minutes, Drain and add to blender with the rest of the ingredients. Add more water only if needed. Add salt and pepper and add zucchini noodles to soup. *Serves 2*

Page | 80

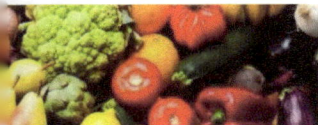

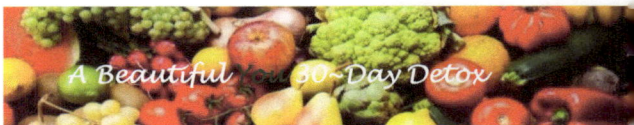

Cream of Spinach Soup

2 cups spinach
½ avocado
½ chopped medium onion
1 chopped celery stalk
1 lime, juiced
½ tsp. cumin
½ tsp. coriander
1 clove garlic
¾ tsp. grey sea salt
1 tsp. miso
1 tbsp. nutritional yeast

Blend all ingredients together until smooth and warm. Serve warm. *Serves 2*

Creamy Carrot Soup

½ cup hazelnuts
1 ½ cups water
3 cups carrots cut into chunks
1 apple, peeled, cored and sliced
1 avocado
1 tbsp. raw honey
1 tsp. ginger
1 tsp. cinnamon
Grey sea salt to taste

Place hazelnuts and water in the food processer and process until smooth. Add remaining ingredients and process until smooth. Salt and pepper to taste. *Serves 4*

Spicy Bok Choy ~ Coconut Soup

4 cups thinly sliced bok choy
6 tbsp. Bragg's Liquid Amino, divided
4 tbsp. sesame oil, divided
1 ½ cups thinly sliced shitake mushrooms
1 tbsp. maple syrup
1 young Thai coconut, both meat and liquid
Water, enough to make 2 ½ cups total when with liquid from the coconut
½ tsp. cumin
½ tsp. turmeric
1 1 – inch piece of ginger, chopped
1 tsp. hot chili garlic sauce
Grey sea salt

Toss bok choy with 3 tbsp. Bragg's Liquid Amino and 2 tbsp. sesame oil. Dehydrate at 115 for 1 hour. If you don't have a dehydrator, then set your oven at the lowest temperature and keep an eye on your bok choy. Toss mushrooms with remaining Bragg's, sesame oil and maple syrup and let marinate for at least one hour. Place coconut flesh, coconut water and water in high speed blender, such as a VitaMix and blend until mixture starts to feel warm.

Page | 81

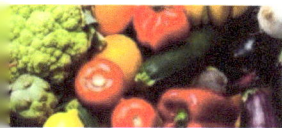

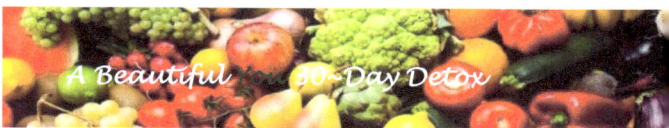

Add cumin, turmeric, ginger, hot chili garlic sauce, salt and pepper and blend until combined. Place in a bowl and add bok choy and mushrooms. Re-heat if desired. *Serves 4*

HOT CHILI GARLIC SAUCE

6 oz. hot chilies, chopped
4 garlic cloves, chopped
½ tsp. grey sea salt
½ tbsp. Bragg's apple cider vinegar

Place all ingredients in food processor and pulse until course. Let stand for 30 minutes to marry flavors. This is HOT, so please use it sparingly!

Raw Tomato Basil Soup

3 medium sized ripe Roma tomatoes, sliced in half
3 sun-dried tomatoes, chopped
2 stalks celery
Pinch onion powder
Pinch garlic powder, I love garlic, so I use a large pinch
½ avocado
1 – 2 sprigs basil
1/8 tsp. dried oregano
Grey sea salt and pepper to taste

Process tomatoes in a high speed blender. Add sun-dried tomatoes and blend until smooth. While blender is going, add the celery, oregano, sea salt, and onion and garlic powders and keep blender going until completely incorporated. Add basil at the end and continue to blend then add the avocado and blend for a few seconds more to combine. Do not over process avocado because it can become discolored. *Serves 4*

Cream of Asparagus Soup

1 bunch raw asparagus
1 ripe avocado
1 liter coconut water
1 cup raw cashews
¼ cup fresh dill
Juice from 1 lemon
1 tsp. tamari
2 garlic cloves
Pinch onion powder
½ tsp black pepper
1 raw, ear fresh corn, kernels removed from cob

Add all ingredients with the exception of the corn and blend. If you can't fit all of the ingredients in your blender, do 2 batches and mix together. Blend until you have your desired texture. Top with fresh corn and serve. *Serves 4*

Vietnamese Pho Soup

4 cups water
2 cups dried shitake
2 tbsp. tamari

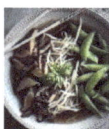

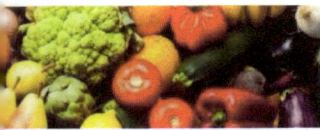

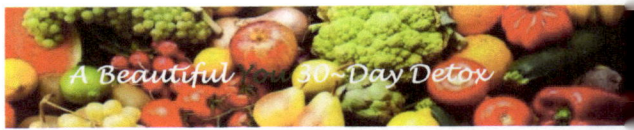

2 tsp. fresh grated ginger
1 tsp. sesame oil
1 – 2 tsp. hot garlic chili sauce
2 cups mung beans sprouts
1 cup snow peas
Sprig fresh basil (for garnish)

Soak mushrooms in water for at least 6 hours. Remove mushrooms from broth and set aside. Strain broth in a bowl and whisk in tamari, ginger, sesame oil and hot garlic chili sauce. Gently warm broth if desired. Cut stems off the mushrooms and thinly slice the caps. Discard stems. Place beansprouts in bowl and pour war broth over them. Top with mushrooms, snow peas and basil. *Serves 4*

Butternut Squash Soup

3 cups butternut squash, peeled and cubed
1 apple
1 avocado
1 tbsp. tamari
2 tbsp. EVOO
½" piece of ginger, minced
1 tsp. grey sea salt
½ tsp cumin
¼ tsp. onion powder
¼ tsp. cinnamon
1 to 1 ½ cups coconut water as needed for the right consistency.

Blend all ingredients with the exception of the avocado in a high speed blender. Add avocado while blender is still blending as this will make the soup nice and creamy. This soup can be served warm or cold. Top with fresh corn and serve. *Serves 4*

Tomato Gazpacho Soup

3 cups ripe Roma tomatoes, chopped
1 cup peeled, chopped cucumber
1 ½ cup red bell pepper
¼ to ½ of a red onion
4 fresh cloves garlic
1 tbsp. about ½ hot green chili
1 tsp. grey sea salt
¼ cup cold water or more for your desired consistency
1/8 tsp. plus 1/8 tbsp. EVOO
¼ cup fresh lemon juice
2 tbsp. stevia in the raw

Add all ingredients to the blender and pulse to desired consistency. To make the chunky mixture and toppings,
2 cups finely diced tomatoes
1 cup finely diced green peppers
1/3 cup about 1 stick finely chopped celery
1 tbsp. EVOO
Pinch of grey sea salt
Toss all ingredients in a bowl with olive oil and sea salt just to bring a nice sheen and to bring out the flavors to the mixture. Add this mixture into the blended mixture and place

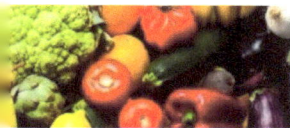

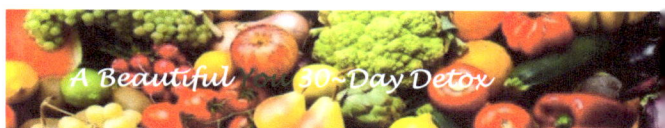

soup in the fridge until completely chilled. Allow a few hours to marry the flavors. *Serves 2 – 4*

Bonus Soup! Raw Dilly Chilled Mango Green Soup

½ cup zucchini
½ cup ripe mango
2 tbsp. fresh dill
½ avocado
Pinch grey sea salt
1 – 2 cups coconut water, add slowly and add more for desired texture
1 lime, juiced

Combine all ingredients except lime juice in blender on high until smooth. Enjoy now or serve chilled. If eating the next day, leave lime out. It will be bitter. *Serves 2*

WARM SOUPS

When you blend your hot soup, do it slowly and work in batches if need be. Be careful not bot burn yourself or risk the steam blowing the lid off of your blender.

Hot Butternut Squash Soup

1 tbsp. EVOO
1 garlic clove, thinly sliced
½ yellow onion
1 large butternut squash
2 red apples
1 avocado
2 cups water
¼ tsp. grey sea salt
¼ tsp. freshly ground black pepper
½ tsp fresh thyme

Preheat oven to 400°F. cut the squash lengthwise in half. Remove seeds and discard. Place squash halves cut side up in baking pan, cover with foil and bake for 45 to 50 minutes. Set aside to cool. Meanwhile, heat olive oil in a medium nonstick sauce pan over medium heat. Add garlic and onion and sauté for just a minute until fragrant. Add apple cook for 4 more minutes or until tender. Add water, salt and pepper and bring to boil. Lower to a simmer and cover. Cover for 8 minutes until tender. When the butternut squash is cool, scoop out into a blender and pour the cooked apples and onion mixture into the blender along with the thyme. Blend until smooth and add avocado and blend for a minute. *Serves 4*

Sea Vegetable Soup with Miso and Shitake Mushrooms

5 cups water

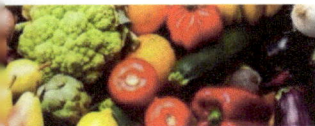

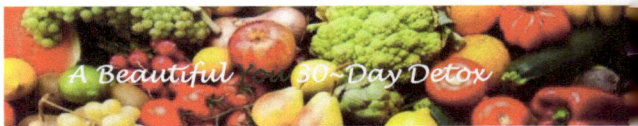

1 strip kombu, hijiki or other sea vegetable. Available at Whole Foods Store or Japanese grocery store.
1 cup chopped bok choy
½ cup chopped carrots
6 – 8 dried shitake mushrooms
5 tsp. miso of your choice

Pour boiling water over mushrooms and let soak for at least an hour before starting. Rinse sea veggies in cold water for 10 minutes. (If using arame, don't soak) Wipe with a towel to remove excess sodium. Fill pot with the water. Cut the sea veggies into small strips and add to pot. Bring the water to boil. Add the carrots, cover the pot and turn the heat to medium-low. Simmer for about 10 minutes. By now, mushrooms should soaked. Strain broth from mushroom over the pot. Remove a little broth to mix with the miso to form a puree. Place the miso mixture into the pot and simmer for 2 – 3 minutes. Never boil your miso because it will kill the beneficial bacteria. Add greens and simmer for 2 more minutes. *Serves 4*

Food for the Soul Soup

1 tbsp. EVOO
1 large Spanish onion, chopped
2 large carrots, peeled and sliced
2 large zucchini, sliced
2 stalks celery, sliced
1 large ripe avocado
2 tbsp. minced fresh dill
1 large handful of spinach
1 tsp. grey sea salt
1/8 tsp. red pepper flakes
4 cups water

Sauté onion, carrots, and celery for 3 minutes. Add rest of ingredients except avocado. Bring to boil and cook for at least 17 to 20 minutes. Place in blender and blend until smooth. Add avocado and blend for 30 seconds or until blended in. *Serves 4*

Hindi Sweet Potato Soup

1 tbsp. EVOO
1 large Spanish onion, chopped
4 sweet potatoes, chopped
2 parsnips, chopped
1 ripe avocado
1 garlic clove
1 tsp. curry powder
¼ tsp. cinnamon
1 can light coconut milk or use rice milk
2 cups coconut water
1 cup spinach
Grey sea salt and pepper to taste
¼ tsp tabasco or cayenne pepper for a little kick

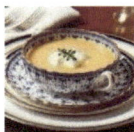

In large soup pot, heat oil over medium heat and add onions, sweet potatoes, chopped parsnip and garlic and sauté for 5 minutes. Add rest of ingredients, including water to the pot with the exception of the spinach and avocado and bring to boil. Reduce heat and

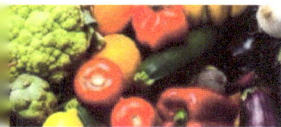

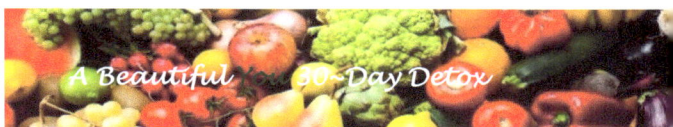

simmer until all veggies are cooked thoroughly, for about 30 minutes. Puree in blender and throw in spinach and avocado at the end. *Serves 4*

Cream of Cauliflower Soup

1 tbsp. EVOO
1 medium head of cauliflower, chopped
1 sweet onion
3 cloves garlic, minced
3 cups filtered water
1 cup kale, chopped
3 tbsp. organic miso paste
1 ripe avocado
2 tbsp. fresh basil
1 tsp. grey sea salt
Chopped parsley to garnish

Roughly chop onions and garlic. Add to large soup pot with olive oil and sauté for 5 minutes on medium high heat. Add cauliflower to soup pot with onions and garlic. Cover with filtered water and cook for about 30 minutes or until cauliflower is tender. When cauliflower is fully cooked, use either an immersion blender or transfer to a high speed blender. Blend and add avocado. Return mixture to the pot and add miso paste fresh basil and chopped kale. Let the warm soup wilt the kale and serve. *Serves 4*

Savory Red Lentil Soup

1 tbsp. EVOO
2 medium onions, chopped
2 stalks celery, chopped
4 garlic cloves, chopped
3 carrots, peeled and chopped
4 tomatoes, chopped
5 cups vegetable broth, (organic yeast free)
5 cups filtered water
2 heads kale, torn into bite size pieces
2 tbsp. dark miso
1 tsp. oregano
1 bay leaf
1 tsp. red pepper flakes
2 tsp. Bragg's apple cider vinegar
2 cups red lentils, rinsed

In a large soup pot, heat olive oil on a low heat and add the onion, celery, garlic and carrots and stir-fry for 10 minutes. Add the tomatoes and stir-fry for 5 more minutes. Add the remaining ingredients except the greens and miso and bring to a boil, uncovered over high heat. When it reaches a boil, cover and turn the heat down to low. Let simmer for 45 minutes. Add the greens and cook for another 10 minutes. Remove some of the soup broth and add to miso past and whisk together. Add back to pot and simmer for another 2 minutes. *Do not boil. Serves 4*

Ginger ~ Kale Soup with Miso

6 cups coconut water or filtered water

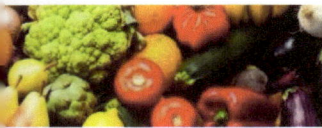

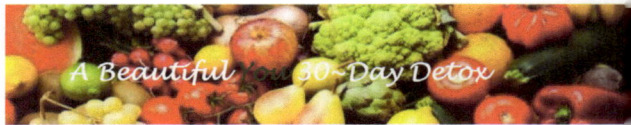

1 bunch kale, de-stemmed, torn into bite size pieces and divided
1 cup sliced carrots
1 tsp. fresh grated ginger
½ avocado
½ cup yellow miso
1 medium leek whites, sliced
Freshly ground pepper (white if you can find it)

Put half the kale and half the ginger into a pot. Bring to a boil, reduce and simmer for 10 minutes. Remove from heat and let cool for 10 minutes. Stir in miso along with the remaining kale, carrots and leeks. Make sure to stir well enough so that the miso is completely dissolved. Garnish with avocado. *Serves 4*

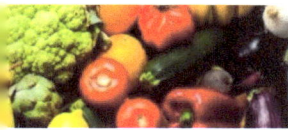

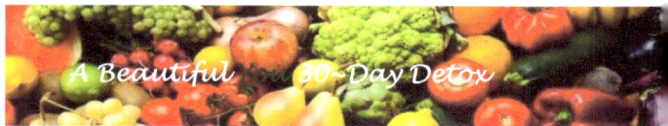

DRESSINGS

Make sure to store your dressings in the fridge for up to 3 days in airtight containers.

Tahini Dressing

½ cup tahini
½ cup cilantro
1 garlic clove, minced
1 tbsp. tamari
Juice of 1 lemon
¼ - ½ cup water

Whisk or blend all ingredients together. Add more water for desired consistency.

Honey Lemon Dressing

2 tsp. fresh lemon juice
1 tsp finely grated lemon zest
1 tbsp. honey
½ tsp. chopped basil
¼ cup EVOO
Grey sea salt and pepper to taste

In a small bowl, whisk together lemon juice with zest, honey and basil. Slowly whisk in the olive oil and add sea salt and pepper to taste

Oil and Vinegar with a Kick

2 – 3 tbsp. Bragg's apple cider vinegar
1 tbsp. Dijon mustard
¾ tsp. cumin
¼ to ½ cup EVOO
Dash of tabasco sauce
Grey sea salt and pepper to taste

Whisk together all ingredients in a bowl except the oil. Then slowly incorporate the oil as needed until it reaches its desired dressing consistency.

Pineapple ~ Ginger Dressing

1 cup pineapple, chopped
½" piece of ginger
½ cup water
Combine all ingredients in a blender.

Simple Miso Dressing

1 tbsp. miso paste
Juice of 1 lemon
1/8 tsp. garlic powder

Page | 88

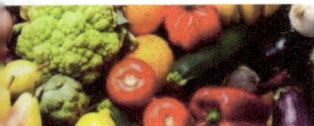

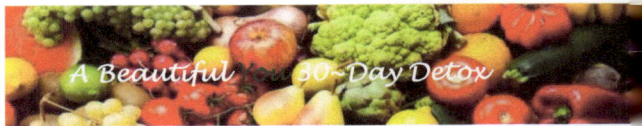

1/8 tsp. dried Italian seasoning
1 tsp. EVOO

Whisk all ingredients together. *Serves 1*

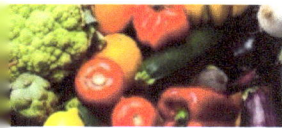

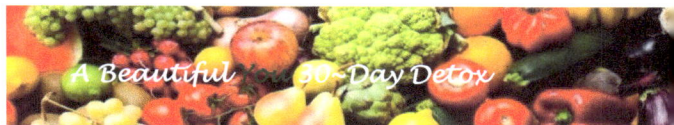

SNACKS

Trail Mix

½ cup dried cranberries
½ cup dried, unsweetened pineapple
½ cup chopped, toasted sunflower seeds
½ cup toasted pumpkin seed
¼ cup raisins, (omit if you're on a candida diet, or need to be on a low sugar diet)
1/8 cup unsweetened coconut

Combine all ingredients and enjoy! *Serves 4*

Stuffed Fig or Date

1 fig or date
1 – 2 tbsp. pumpkin seed butter or sun butter
1 tsp. banana, mashed
Dash raw honey
Stevia in the raw (optional)

Combine nut butter with banana and set aside. Empty fig or date, then stuff with nut mixture and sprinkle with cinnamon and drizzle raw honey. *Serves 1*

Kale Chips

1 bunch kale, de-stemmed and leaves torn into 2" pieces
2 tbsp. EVOO
1 tbsp. fresh lime juice
¼ cup sesame seeds
Grey sea salt

Preheat oven to 200°F for 1 hour. In large bowl, drizzle kale with lime juice and sesame seeds. Season with grey sea salt. Toss until evenly coated. Transfer to a rimmed baking sheet and bake for 30 minutes. Remove from oven and, using a spatula, flip kale leaves over. Return to oven and continue cooking until kale is dry and crisp, 20 – 25 minutes. Let cool completely. Store in airtight container for up to 3 days.

Sweet Potato Delight

Bake sweet potato at 350°F for an hour. Split down the middle and add ½ tsp coconut oil, cinnamon, raw honey and sliced bananas if you need a sweet pick-me-up.

That Chocolate Thing You Do

2 tbsp. unsweetened coconut
2 tbsp. raw cacao
2 tbsp. goji berries
2 tbsp. dried cranberries
2 tbsp. raisins

Mix all ingredients together for an afternoon pick-me-up.

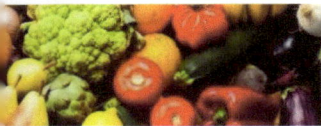

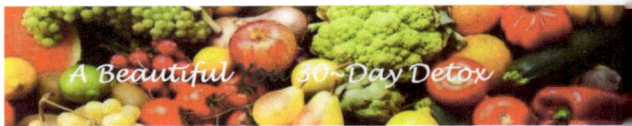

Fancy Avocado

Top ½ avocado with Mediterranean Spiced Sea Salt, a pinch of garlic and a dash of cayenne.

Delectable Sweet Potato

Season ½ baked sweet potato with garlic powder, grey sea salt and a drizzle of tahini dressing.

The Beverage Center

Pick your favorite juice recipe and add unsweetened coconut milk, vanilla & cinnamon.

Banana Ecstasy

Slice a banana lengthways down the middle and top with tahini or sun butter & sprinkle with shredded coconut and raisins.

Purse Treat

Combine a handful of seeds with your favorite fresh fruit

Collard Wraps with Turmeric Spread

1 cup coconut flesh
1/3 cup coconut water
1 garlic clove
Juice from ½ lime
1 tsp. maple syrup
½ tsp coriander
Pinch of grey sea salt

Blend all ingredients in high speed blender until smooth and set aside for flavors to marry.
For the wraps you'll need:
4 collard leaves
½ red bel pepper, cut into thin strips
1 carrot, cut into thin strips
1 cup cherry tomatoes, halved
Place filling ingredients onto collard leaf and top with dressing. Roll and cut in half. *Serves 4*

Sun ~ Dried Tomatoes Dressed in Green

1 cup cashews
½ cup pine nuts
¼ cup pumpkin seeds
¼ cup sun-dried tomatoes, softened
Juice from ½ lemon
½ shallot, about 2 tbsp.
1 garlic clove
Pinch grey sea salt
1 cup fresh pea pods, split

Soak cashews, pine nuts and pumpkin seeds until soft (about 2 hours). Combine with the rest of the ingredients except pea pods in the food processor and process until smooth. Pipe

Page | 91

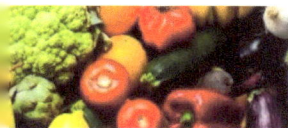

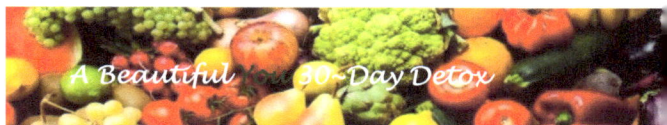

into split pea pods. You'll have left over spread, so store it in the fridge for at least 3 – 4 days. You can use also use the rest of to spread over raw pasta. *Serves 2 – 4*

Zucchini Steamboats

2 small zucchini
1 ripe avocado
¼ cup adzuki beans
1 tbsp. tahini
½ tsp. garlic powder
½ tsp. grey sea salt
Juice of ½ lime or lemon
TOPPINGS
Green bell pepper
Green olives
Basil

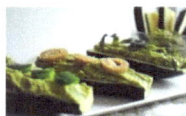

In food processor, blend together, avocado, adzuki beans, tahini, water, garlic powder, grey sea salt and lemon or lime juice. Make sure to scrape down the sides to keep the consistency. Don't leave any of the adzuki beans chunky.
Prepare zucchini by rinsing and drying and trimming off the ends. Slice in half lengthwise and use a melon scooper or a small spoon to scrape out the inside. Fill the inside, hollowed out portion of the zucchini with the mixture and smooth out. Top with green olives and sliced green peppers. Do a chiffonade cut on the basil and ribbon it on top. *Serves 4*

Scrumptious Poppers

The day before, make the eggplant bacon in the dehydrator. If you don't have one, use the lowest setting in your oven.
1 eggplant
2 tbsp. EVOO
¼ water
1 tsp. smoked paprika
½ ground chipotle peppers
2 tbsp. maple syrup

Using a vegetable or mandolin, slice eggplant into strips about 1/8" thick and set aside. Place in the above marinade and soak for a good 2 hours. Dehydrate at 116 for at least 12 hours.
Day of:
FILLING
1 ½ cup pine nuts, pre-soaked for 4 – 5 hours
½ cup pumpkin seeds pre-soaked for 4 – 5 hours
½ cup cashews pre-soaked for 4 – 5 hours
Juice from 1 ½ lemons
2 tbsp. nutritional yeast
1 tbsp. smoked paprika
Pinch grey sea salt
½ red pepper

Place all ingredients in food processor until smooth. Halve 10 red jalapeno peppers, remove seeds and fill with filling and top with eggplant bacon. *Serves 4-6*

Lemony Cups

2 cups finely grated carrots

Page | 92

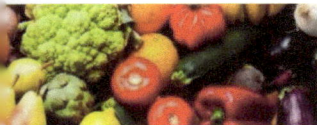

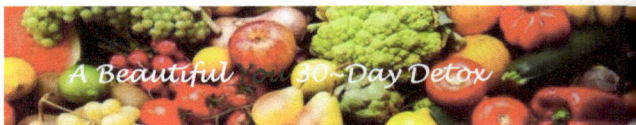

1 tbsp. lemon juice
1 tsp. EVOO
Stevia or maple syrup
¼ of a yellow bell pepper
4 lemons halved

In a small mixing bowl, toss the carrots yellow bell pepper, lemon juice, zest and oil. Taste and sweeten if desired. Fill lemon halves with carrot mixture. *Serves 4*

Dilly Stuffed Tomatoes

4 medium tomatoes
½ cup celery, diced
½ cup water chestnuts, sliced
1/3 cup scallions, thinly sliced
1/3 cup sunflower seeds
¼ cup pumpkin seeds
Grey sea salt to taste
DILL DRESSING
1 cup cashews, soaked overnight
½ cup water
3 tbsp. Bragg's apple cider vinegar
2 tsp. dried mustard
2 tsp. lemon juice
Grey sea salt and pepper to taste
1 tsp minced garlic
4 tsp. fresh dill, chopped

Place all dressing ingredients in high speed blender and blend until smooth. Cut off tops of tomatoes and scoop out the insides. Dice tops and set aside. Toss together tomato tops, celery, water chestnuts and seeds. At this point, add the sea salt and pepper or mix in 2 – 3 tbsp. of the dill dressing. Fill tomatoes and top with a spot of dressing. *Serves 4*

Tea Sandwiches in the Raw

2 beets, 1 red and 1 golden
1 cucumber (half sliced, half diced)
1 cup pine nuts
¼ cup pumpkin seeds

1 tbsp. nutritional yeast
½ cup thinly sliced scallions
1 cup diced cucumber (from the cucumber above)
1 tbsp. tarragon
Grey sea salt and pepper to taste

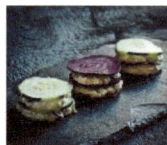

Slice the beets and half the cucumbers into rounds. Place pine nuts, pumpkin seeds, nutritional yeast, and water and lemon juice in food processor. Process until very smooth. In a small bowl, stir in scallions, diced cucumbers and the tarragon. Salt and pepper to taste. Construct you tea sandwiches in any fashion you like. *Serves 2 - 4*

Ants on a Log

2 tbsp. tahini
A drizzle of honey

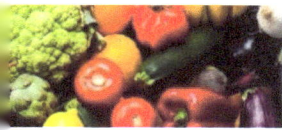

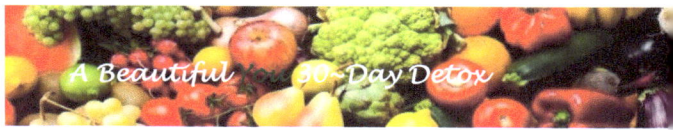

1 celery stalk
¼ cup raisins

Mix honey and tahini well. Put mixture inside the celery stalk and sprinkle with raisins.
Serves 1

Banana ~ Tahini Celery Delight

¼ piece of banana
2 tbsp. raw honey
2 tbsp. tahini
1 celery
¼ cup raisins

Mash banana well and mix with tahini and honey. Put mixture in celery and sprinkle with raisins. *Serves 1*

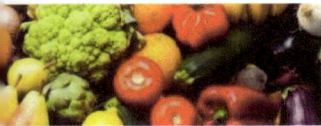

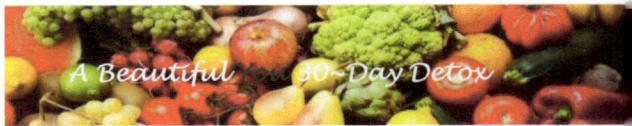

TRANSITION RECIPES

SuperFood Quinoa Breakfast Bowl

½ cooked quinoa, (follow the package directions before making this recipe)
1/8 cup pumpkin seeds
4 tbsp. flax meal
½ cup almond milk
¼ cup frozen blueberries
¼ cup sliced strawberries
Drizzle of honey or maple syrup to taste

Combine all ingredients in a bowl and serve warm. *Serves 1 – 2*

Organic Breakfast Bowl

2 apples or pears, peeled and shredded
1 banana, sliced
2 2bsp. Hemp seeds
¼ tsp. cinnamon
1 tbsp. raisins, currants or 1 – 2 medjool dates, chopped
Juice of ½ lemon
¼ cup coconut milk or rice milk

Add the apples and bananas to a bowl. Mix in all ingredients. Pour milk over the mixture and serve. *Serves 2*

Italian Hummus

1 can organic cannellini beans
¼ cup tahini
2 oz. EVOO
½ red pepper
½ - 1 tsp. grey sea salt
1 ½ tsp. cumin
1 garlic clove, mashed
¼ cup fresh lemon juice
Dash of cayenne
Warm filtered water (to loosen the consistency of your hummus)

Process all ingredients in a blender or food processor. With processor running add warm water to the consistency that you desire. Put in a serving bowl and top with chopped parsley and sprinkle on some paprika and cumin. *Serves 2 – 4*

Moroccan Quinoa Salad

1 1/3 cups cooked quinoa
1 stick cinnamon, about 2"
2 tsp. coriander seeds
1 tsp. cumin seeds
2 tbsp. EVOO

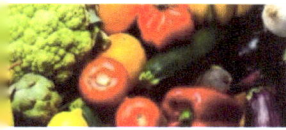

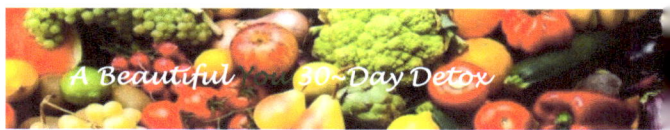

1 small onion, finely chopped
2 garlic cloves, finely chopped
½ tsp. ground turmeric
Pinch cayenne
1 tbsp. lemon juice
1/3 sugar free golden raisins
3 ripe Roma tomatoes
3 oz. cucumber, about 1/3 piece
4 scallions
3 tbsp. chopped fresh cilantro
Grey sea salt and pepper to taste

In a small pan, heat the cinnamon stick, coriander and cumin seeds. Over high heat, cook until seeds pop and smell fragrant, carefully watching so as not to burn. Remove from heat and grind in a spice grinder then add the rest of the spices to the mixture and set aside. In a clean pan, heat oil and add the onions. Cook over low heat for 7 – 8 minutes until slightly browned. Add garlic and cook for another minute. Add spices and cook for another minute. Remove from heat and add lemon juice. Add this mixture to the quinoa and mix thoroughly, making sure all the quinoa is coated. Add remaining ingredients and salt and pepper to taste. *Serves 4*

SuperFood Goji Balls

3 cups raw organic oat flakes
¾ cup pumpkin seeds
¾ cup sunflower seeds
6 medjool dates
½ cup cacao nibs, ground
1/3 cup almond flour
¼ cup maple syrup
½ cup melted coconut oil, melted
½ cup almond butter
½ cup goji berries

Mix oats, seeds, and almond flour in a large bowl and set aside. In a food processor, chop dates. Place dates in a separate bowl and add agave and melted maple syrup and coconut oil. Massage and mix well. Pour wet ingredients into the same bowl as the dry and mix well. Add goji berries then form into 1" balls. Chill to set.

Butternut Squash Bowl

1 butternut squash
1 tbsp. coconut oil
¼ tsp. cinnamon
1 avocado, diced
1 mango, diced
1 cup broccoli, chopped and steamed
¼ tsp garlic powder
Juice of ½ lime
Grey sea salt to taste

Preheat oven to 400°F. cut squash lengthwise in half and remove the seeds. Place squash halves cut side up on baking pan. Cover with foil and bake for 45 – 50 minutes. Set aside to cool. Once cooled, cube and place in a bowl. Add coconut oil and cinnamon and let it

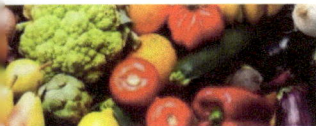

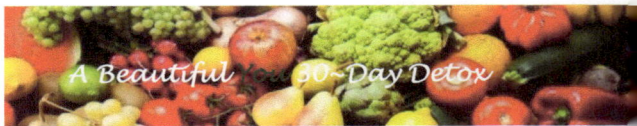

melt throughout. Add broccoli and mango along with the lime juice to the butternut squash and mix well. Add avocado and garlic powder to the dish and combine. *Serves 4*

Asparagus ~ Quinoa Risotto

1 cup quinoa
1 shallot, finely chopped
½ tbsp. EVOO
1 cup light coconut milk
1 cup asparagus, chopped
½ red pepper, chopped
Juice of 1 lemon
Pinch of cayenne
½ tsp thyme
Grey sea salt and pepper to taste

Cook quinoa according to package directions and set aside. In a sauce pan, heat olive oil and sauté shallot. Add shallot to quinoa and begin adding coconut milk. Add ¼ cup at a time, stirring all the while until the quinoa soaks it up. You might not need the full cup. While you're doing this, steam your asparagus and red pepper. When they are tender, add them to the quinoa and coconut milk. Stir in juice from lemon and add the thyme, cayenne, salt and pepper. *Serves 2*

Moroccan Spiced Bowl

2 tbsp. EVOO
¾ cup quinoa
1 ¼ cup water
4 tbsp. lemon flavored oil or EVOO
1 tbsp. lemon juice
3 tbsp. vinegar
1 tbsp. honey
1 tsp. garam masala
1 tsp. coriander
½ tsp. mustard
8 oz. canned kidney beans
8 oz. canned garbanzo beans
2 shallots, chopped
4 scallions, trimmed and sliced
½ cup pine nuts
¾ cup golden sugar free raisins
1 tbsp. chopped mint

Rinse quinoa thoroughly the night before so that it could dry in the fridge. Heat oil in a large pan and add quinoa. Cook for 3 minutes, stirring over a low heat. Pour in the water and bring to a boil, then lower the heat, cover and simmer for 35 minutes. Remove from heat a strain. Rinse under cold running water and drain well. Set aside. In a large bowl, mix together the lemon flavored or EVOO, vinegar, lemon juice and honey. Add garam masala, coriander and mustard and mix well. Add quinoa and mix well. Rinse and drain beans then add them to the bowl with the shallots, scallions, pine nuts, golden raisins and mint. *Serves 4*

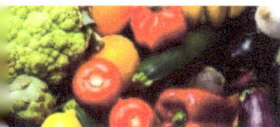

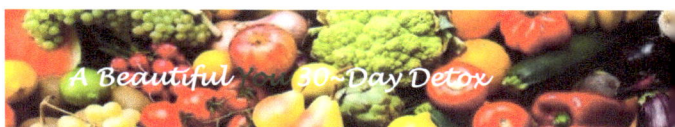

DESSERTS

Raw Pudding

1 avocado
2 bananas
1 cup almond milk
1 zucchini, chopped
1 tbsp. raw cacao powder
1 tbsp. raw honey

Place all ingredients in a high speed blender and process until smooth. Put in the fridge until it's cold. *Serves 2*

Creamsicle

2 oranges
1 cup unsweetened almond milk
1 tbsp. ground chia seeds
½ tsp. Vanilla extract
½ tsp almond extract
Squeeze of lime juice
Squeeze of lemon juice

Place all ingredients in blender and blend well. Place into Popsicle molds and freeze.

Spice of Life Oatmeal Drink

1/3 cup raw oats, soaked overnight and rinsed
1 ½ cups almond milk, room temp.
1 banana
2 medjool dates
Small handful of raisins
½ tbsp. almond butter
¼ tsp. nutmeg
1/8 tsp cinnamon
¼ tsp. ground ginger

Add all ingredients into a high-speed blender and blend until smooth and warm.

Fruity Chia Dessert

2 tbsp. ground chia
1 banana
1 cup strawberries
1 peach, slightly blended
1 cup unsweetened coconut or almond milk
1 tbsp. shredded coconut
1 tbsp. maple syrup

Combine all ingredients in a bowl and chill in the fridge until chia seeds turn into a pudding consistency, for 20 – 30 minutes.

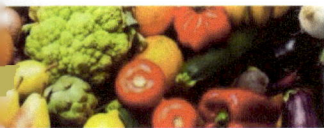

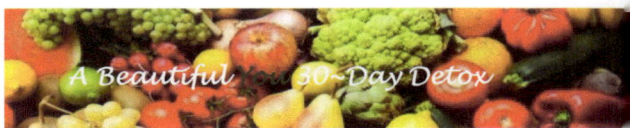

Blackberry Sorbet

½ cups frozen blackberries
¾ cup unsweetened cup almond, coconut, rice or hemp milk
1 tbsp. ground chia seed
2 tbsp. maple syrup
½ tsp. vanilla extract
¼ tsp. almond extract
Squirt of lemon juice

Combine all ingredients in a high speed blender and enjoy!

Mixed Berry Sorbet

4 – 5 cups frozen mixed berries
Juice of one lime
1/3 cup maple syrup
Crushed mint leaves
1 tbsp. chia seed, grounded

Place all ingredients in a blender and pulse until desired consistency. Stir in mint leaves.

Simply Yum Mix – Up

3 tbsp. coconut flakes
1 tbsp. ground flax seed
2 tbsp. frozen blueberries
1 tsp cacao powder
1 tsp. coconut oil
1 tsp. maple syrup
Pinch of salt

Combine all ingredients in a high – speed blender for a really quick dessert that you can throw together so simply!

Your Chocolate Moment

2 bars organic dark chocolate (I like 85% cacao)
1 cup raw almonds, chopped
1 cup unsweetened, shredded coconut
2 tbsp. EVCO
Grey sea salt
Colorful berries for garnish

Break chocolate up into small pieces and melt over a double broiler. I like to use a small sauce pan placed over a larger sauce pan filled with boiling water. Remember – melting chocolate over steam prevents burning. Add chopped almonds, shredded coconut, coconut oil and salt. Stir well. Line a baking sheet with parchment paper or wax paper and drop spoon full of the chocolate mixture about an inch apart on the sheet. Place in the fridge until chilled. *Serves 12*

BONUS DESSERTS – POST TRANSITION GUILTLESS SWEETS

Chocolate Moonlight Guiltless Balls

1 cup walnuts
½ cup Brazil nuts

Page | 99

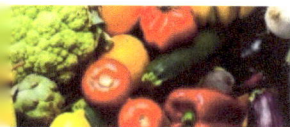

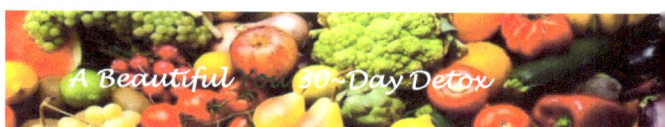

8 medjool dates
¼ cup dried cherries or cranberries
¼ cup dried coconut
2 tbsp. cacao powder
1 tbsp. coconut oil
1 tbsp. raw honey or maple syrup
¼ cup goji berries
Hemp or sesame seeds (to roll your balls into)

Combine all ingredients in a food processor and blend away. You want everything to be combined yet not fully blended. Some chunks are nice. Form into small balls or flatten. Roll in hemp or sesame seeds.

Sleepy Time Milkshake

1 cup almond milk
2 frozen bananas
½ cups frozen strawberries
1 tbsp. raw cacao
2 tbsp. almond butter
4 medjool dates
¼ tsp. cinnamon
Dash of cayenne (optional)

Combine all ingredients in high – speed blender and enjoy!

Yummy Quinoa 'N' Milk

2 cups unsweetened almond milk
2 cups cooked quinoa or millet
2 cups filtered water
1 tsp. maple syrup or stevia
1 tbsp. almond butter
1 banana, chopped
Hemp seeds (optional)

Combine quinoa or millet with water in a saucepan on high heat until boiling. Cover, reduce heat to low and simmer for 15 minutes. After 15 minutes, add almond milk, syrup or sweetener of your choice, stir to combine. Place in a bowl and top with almond butter and banana. You can, if desired, sprinkle with hemp seeds. *Serves 2*

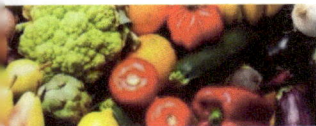

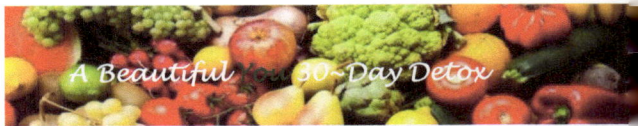

Chapter 14 – Articles You'll Need Along the Way

JOURNALING – WRITE YOURSELF THIN TO THE BODY YOU DESIRE!

Success is attained when we not only want something deep in our hearts, and souls, as well in the foreground of our mind, but when we write it down…Every day you are going to be very clear on what your intentions and goals are. Clarity not only come when you think these things through, but you make them a part of your daily lives when you write them down.

> "Setting goals is the first step in turning the invisible into the visible."
> ~ Tony Robbins

PRE – TOX

Write down your intentions for your Pre – Tox:

_____
_____
_____
_____
____

Reflect:

1. What's exciting you? Write it down.
2. What rites will you begin your day with and include into your life?
   - Drink more water
   - Drink your Lemon/Lime regimen
   - Do one of the Detox Feel Greats
   - Breathing or Meditation
   - Slow down on the consumption of processed foods and coffee
3. Do an evening report: Write down an aspect of your Pre – Tox day that made you feel good. What gave you that feeling of excitement, what empowered you or gave you strength for that day. Write down in your journal what happened.

_____
_____
_____

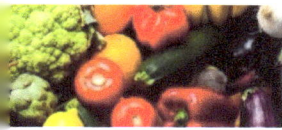

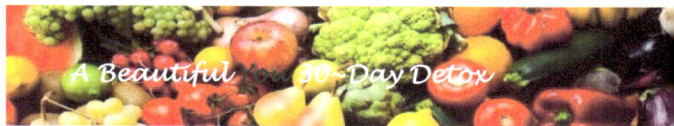

Days 1 – 30:

1. When you begin, using whatever form you like best (notebook, computer, etc…), Journaling what your feelings are having each morning helps you to reflect on your day and what lies ahead. Remember, this is truly a productive process that will set you on the path of victory!

   Think about what you're looking forward to in your daily detox experience. Include things you've chosen to do for YOU. Things like:

   a. Journaling
   b. Eating healing, whole foods
   c. Doing your daily "body check – in" Am I satiated? Am I feeling loved? What am I feeling in my body both physically and emotionally?
   d. Do at least one of the Detox Feel Greats like tongue scraping, hot towel scrub or dry skin brushing
   e. Attaining some me or alone time to devote to yourself
   f. Do your daily encouragements
   g. Drink your lemon water and healing regimens
   h. Have fun, laugh it up and imagine your success all day every day

2. Remember, each night before going to bed, take another couple of minutes to journal your feelings. How did your day go? Pay attention to the following about your body:
   a. Your Energy Levels
   b. Your Sleep Patterns
   c. Your Digestion
   d. Bowel Movements
   e. Moods & Cravings
   f. Hunger Level
   g. Weight Loss

TRANSITION DAYS

While preparing to complete your Detox, it's important to get really clear on what worked for you. Keep in mind that weight loss and detox are not about feeling deprived. Rather, they're about feeling whole and complete from the foods that you choose to eat, the life

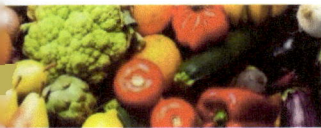

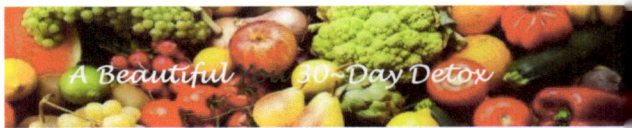

you choose to live and the people you choose to be in your life. This is a great time to look over your Journal from your Detox and see what you've learned from it.

You're almost finished, so let's make sure that you're on track. One wonderful project to create while on your program is a Big Picture Vision Board. This will help you stay on track and make your path clearer.

What is a Big Picture Vision Board?

A Big Picture Vision Board, also referred to as a treasure map, is a simple and fun way to catch all the dreams you have for yourself and your life and turn them into a reality.

A big picture vision board is made from pictures cut from magazines, printed images from the internet and/or photos from our own life that inspires you to be the best version of yourself. Any picture that moves and inspires you toward your goal is a must have for your big picture board. You'll gather all these images and display them together. Your big picture board will be your personal reminder that YOU created an outline for your life, and you do it on a daily basis.

To start your big picture vision board, you'll need to:

1. Be clear on what you desire
2. Be clear on what truly inspires you

To create your big picture vision board:

Get yourself a large poster board or magnetic board. Use magnets, pushpins, tape or glue to display all of the images and pictures that you gather. Now you have a positive expression of your thoughts, goals, inspirations, ideas and ideals.

NOW YOU'RE READY TO START ESTABLISHING YOUR GOALS!

Page | 103

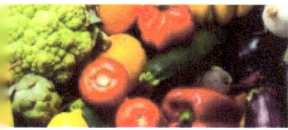

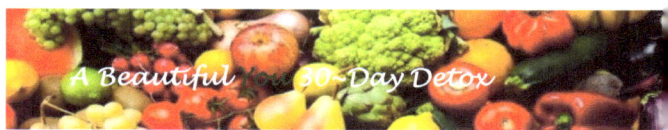

YOUR DAILY MOTIVATION FOR DETOX & WEIGHT LOSS

20 Lifestyle Changes To Help You Ditch Dieting Forever!

1. Cherish yourself.
2. Seek out ways to be truly good to yourself every chance you get.
3. Follow your program to reduce stress. Stress reduction results in the release of toxins and weight loss.
4. Eat purely.
5. Get enough rest.
6. Make time for yourself
7. Get support from family and friends.
8. Drink 80 oz. of lemon water per day.
9. Eat foods with no hormones. Hormones may interfere with your metabolism and/or weight loss.
10. Pay attention to your body and make sure that you are getting enough nutrition by eating healthy foods.
11. Practice proper portion control.
12. Raise your heart rate and keep in mind that exercise provides not only physical results, but also greatly improves your mental capacity.
13. Get rid of the processed foods.
14. Stay positive.
15. Eat foods that promote good health and healing.
16. Create a book of pictures that motivate you and refer to it when you need to be uplifted.
17. Say your daily assertions.
18. Dance at least once a day.
19. Hug yourself at least once a day.
20. Remember, we're not perfect but in the meantime, practice feeling calm.

21 Daily Assertions To Love Yourself Into The Body You Long For!

"It's never just about the food on your plate: Love yourself and the body you deserve and want is yours for the taking"

1. I am loving towards all people and I know that what I'm giving out will be returned to me twice over because I love myself.
2. In my world, I only attract loving people that mirror what and who I am.
3. I am open and receptive to all good and abundance that God has to give me.
4. Today is a lovely day. Blessings come to me in expected and unexpected ways.

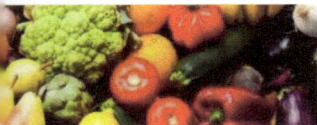

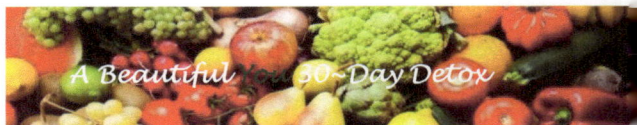

5. I assist my body in a loving way to attain perfect health.

6. When your view of life changes, so does your reality.

7. I shall aspire to share from my heart, the goodness that is within me, striving to be oneness with my creator and lovingly sharing with my fellow man what is required of me to share with them. I will happily and lovingly co-exist with my fellow man and be as innocent as a dove, mild as a lamb and peaceable as the Lord.

8. I consciously commit to flexibility and detachment.

9. I allow myself and those around me to be themselves, without imposing my views or ideals on them.

10. I release need for judgment and criticism.

11. If I see myself becoming argumentative, I take a deep breath and come to a more centered place.

12. I can accomplish anything that I set my mind to with prayer and supplication with ease and comfort.

13. Being me isn't risky. It's my ultimate truth and I live it fearlessly.

14. I inherited infinite patience when it comes to fulfilling my dreams.

15. I'd rather be loathed for what I am than loved for what I'm not.

16. The right conditions along with the right people are already here and will show up on time.

17. Beginning here and now, I'm willing to attract all that I desire.

18. I have access to an unlimited wealth of support. My strength comes from my relationship to my source of being.

19. All is well in my life and I trade love and acceptance with life.

20. I have high self – esteem as I respect myself.

21. **I am truly loved!**

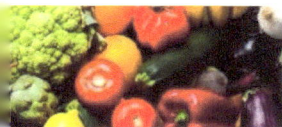

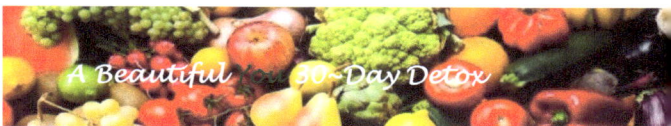

LOW GLYCEMIC FOODS

The tables below will give you an idea of where food falls on the glycemic index. Remember, this chart is **prefect for you during your Post – Tox.** Be balanced where your meals are concerned and keep an eye on your blood sugar. Pay special attention to the last chart of sweeteners. By nature of the foods, all fats and proteins are low glycemic. Always remember that just because a food is low glycemic doesn't mean it's right for your unique body. During your Post – Tox days, pay special attention to your body and how you're feeling.

LOW GLYCEMIC CARBS/FIBER	HIGH GLYCEMIC CARBS/FIBER
100% whole, unprocessed grains ➢ Quinoa ➢ Barley, faro, ancient grains ➢ Brown rice ➢ Sprouted grains ➢ Whole grain pasta cooked al dente	white carbs * White Bread * White rice * White Flour * White tortillas * White pasta * Enriched flour
All raw veggies and most cooked veggies	Cooked corn, cooked carrots, potatoes
Most fruits	Fruit juice
Sea veggies, like seaweed	Bananas, pineapple, mango, watermelon
Sweet potatoes, yams, small potatoes with skin	Corn, tortilla chips, potato chips, most crackers
Rolled or steel cut oats, Kashi Go-Lean cereal	Instant oatmeal, most cereals
Most whole, close to nature foods	Most instant, highly processed foods

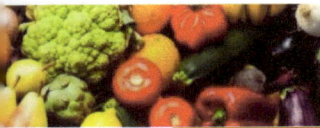

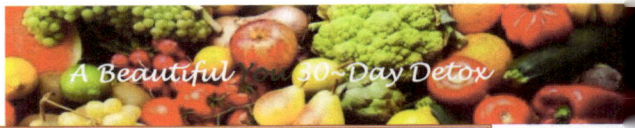

HEALTHY FATS	LESS SUITABLE FATS
OILS: ♥ Extra Virgin Olive Oil ♥ Cold Pressed Flax Oil ♥ Macadamia Nut Oil ♥ Avocado Oil ♥ Coconut Oil	**OILS:** • Peanut Oil • Vegetable Oil • Canola Oil • Soybean Oil • Buy Organic if using these oils as they are highly genetically modified in our country.
NUTS: Always try and eat raw, it's best ♥ Walnuts ♥ Pecans ♥ Pine Nuts ♥ Cashews…they aren't as good for you as almonds and walnuts, but ok in moderation.	Peanuts and peanut butter should be eaten in moderation, they're heavily processed in the U S and aren't really that good for you. Always buy organic over commercial brands. Animal fat in general is saturated fat, and this is what we want you to be mindful of, especially in red meat. If you must have it, limit yourself to it once or twice a month.
SEEDS: Always go for the raw seeds ♥ Hulled Sunflower Seeds ♥ Pumpkin Seeds ♥ Flax Seeds, always ground them, they absorb better ♥ Chia Seeds **SALMON**	**CHEESE:** • Avoid heavily processed cheeses and all cheeses in mass consumption. • Use cheese only as a condiment and not the main dish • Goat's cheeses or milks • Sheep's milk i.e. feta, pecorino Romano and real parmesan • Unpasteurized (Raw) chees is easier to digest because it contains enzymes. DO NOT ENGEST WHILE PREGNANT!

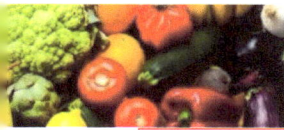

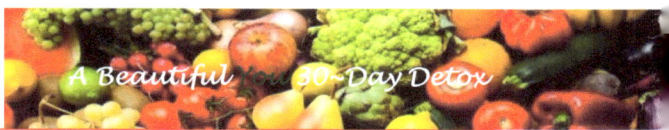

HEALTHY PROTEINS	LESS SUITABLE PROTEINS
PLANTS: ♥ Hemp Seeds ♥ Beans, (Black, White, Navy, Kidney, Pinto, etc. ♥ Lentils ♥ Peas ♥ Edamame (Soy Beans) ♥ Nuts & Seeds…Almonds mostly ♥ Sprouts **ANIMAL:** ♥ Plain Greek Yogurt ♥ Salmon ♥ Tuna ♥ Most caught wild fish ♥ Organic turkey or chicken whole breasts. NO DELI MEATS! ♥ Pork Tenderloin, only in moderation ♥ 1 – 2 Free Range Organic Eggs a day	**MEATS & DAIRY** Meats and dairy should always be eaten in moderation and should always be organic. Lean chicken and turkey is ok, though I'm not a big proponent of meat, so be sure it's organic and not charred because charred meat can cause cancer. Lean pork is an alright option, just don't buy the highly processed breakfast sausages and other processed pork products. Choose plain Greek yogurt. You can add natural sweeteners to it to make it taste delicious. Choose wild caught fish, they're higher in omega-3 fatty acids. If you feel the need to eat meat, opt for game meat because it's very lean and natural, may be a little gamey. Duck, Cornish game hen and other less common meats are ok in moderation too.
SUITABLE SUGARS	LESS SUITABLE SUGARS
♥ Stevia ♥ Agave Nectar Syrup ♥ Raw Honey ♥ Grade B Pure Maple Syrup, limit your intake ♥ Dates and Date Paste ♥ Fructose ♥ Brown Rice Syrup	**THESE AREN'T RECOMMENDED** • All artificial sweeteners • Splenda, Nutra-Sweet, Equal, etc. • All white sugar • High – Fructose Corn Syrup • Sugar in the Raw/Brown Sugar (High glycemic, but better than white sugar because it has some nutrients.)

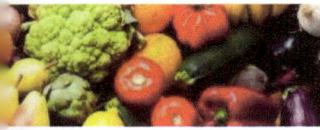

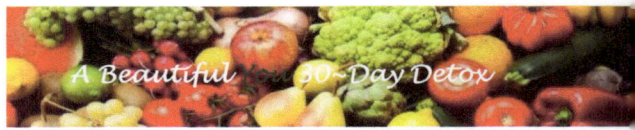

SHOPPING LIST

FRUITS:

Avocados
Bananas
Blackberries
Blueberries
Coconuts
Grapefruits
Green Apples
Kiwis
Lemons
Limes
Mangos
Oranges
Pineapples
Raspberries
Strawberries

_____
_____
_____
_____

VEGETABLES:

Arugula
Basil
Beets
Brussels Sprouts
Butter Lettuce
Carrots
Cauliflower
Celery
Cherry Tomatoes
Corn
Frisee (opt.)
Jicama
Kale
Lettuce Leaves
Onions (red & yellow)
Raw veggies of choice
Red Bell Pepper
Scallions
Shallots
Snow Peas
Spinach
Sprouts

Sun – Dried Tomatoes
Tomatoes
Water Chestnuts
Yellow Squash
Zucchini

_____
_____
_____
_____

PROTEINS:

Ground Chia Seeds
Pumpkin Seeds

FROZEN FOODS:

Blackberries
Blueberries
Cherries
Mixed Berries

_____
_____
_____

CONDIMENTS:

Agave
Coconut Oil
Dijon Mustard
Honey, Raw
Miso, Dark & Light
Extra Virgin Olive Oil (EVOO)
Sauerkraut/Kimchee
Sesame Oil
Sesame Seeds
Stevia
Tahini, (Wheat Free)
Tamari

_____
_____
_____

MISCELLANEOUS:

Dried Coconut Flakes
Garlic
Ground Flax Seed
Hemp Seeds
Nutritional Yeast
Pine Nuts
Raw Cacao

_____
_____

BEVERAGES:

Apple Cider Vinegar Bragg
Unsweetened coconut milk
Unsweetened coconut water
Unsweetened Almond Milk
Coffee, organic (option)
Cranberry Concentrate
Hemp and or Rice Milk
Herbal Tea

_____
_____
_____

HERBS & SPICES:

Cayenne Pepper
Cilantro/Sorrel/Mint
Cinnamon
Coriander
Curry Powder
Fennel
Garlic powder
Ginger, Fresh & Ground
Parsley
Peppercorns
Grey Sea Salt

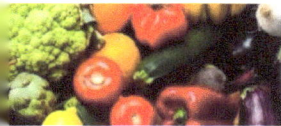

Vanilla Extract

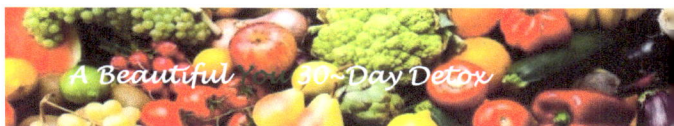

EXTRAS:

_____
_____
_____
_____
_____
_____
_____
_____
_____
_____

**STAGE   ITEMS
FOR   YOUR
TRANSITION:**

Chickpeas
Dates
Flax meal/Chia Meal
Hemp Protein Powder
Raisins / Currants
Scallions
Shredded coconuts
Snap Peas
Sun flower seeds
Sunflower butter
Thyme
Quinoa

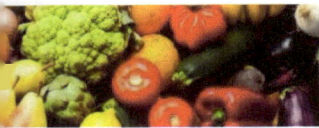

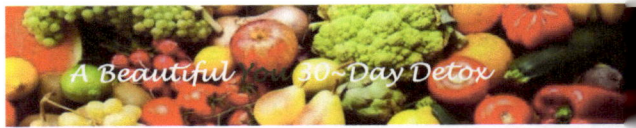

YOUR DAILY FOOD DIARY

Your Daily Food Diary is a powerful tool. By using the Food Diary, you'll begin to see how food affects you both physically and emotionally. Feel free to use the form that I've attached in this book for your convenience. You have several options, you can use a note pad, agenda book or your computer. Make a note on how you feel physically and emotionally before, during and after each meal, snack and beverage. By now, you know how fantabulous it feels to not be bloated, so make a note of this when you add back the foods that were not in the Detox Program.

Good example:

- ➢ Do you feel tired?
- ➢ Do you feel bloated?
- ➢ Do you feel irritated?
- ➢ Does your lower back hurt?
- ➢ Are you constipated?

Get excited for this stage because this is your chance to finally get rid of the diets that don't work, stop counting calories and stop dwelling on carbs, portions and fats as we are simply going to focus on the foods that keep you feeling and looking fantabulous every second of the day.

Even more so in the Transition Diet Stage of your Detox, this process should be fun and informative. Keep in mind that food is not good or bad and your relationship with food is simply defined by what foods fuels your body and gives you endless energy.

Here's a reminder of the reactions and symptoms examples to keep you motivated and on target:

PHYSICAL SYMPTOMS – BODILY SENSATIONS

- Symptoms of imbalance: headaches, stomach pain muscle cramps, muscle cramps, coughing, fatigue, insomnia, restlessness, shakiness, muscle weakness, poor concentration, paleness.
- Symptoms of balance: bright eyes, hunger, stamina, natural deep breathing, energetic, restful sleep, focus, alertness, strength, good attention span, good color.

Page | 111

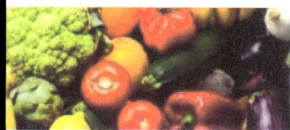

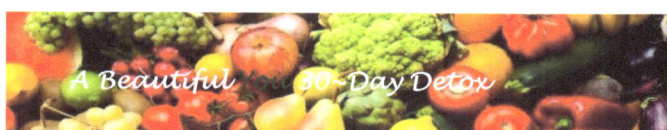

EMOTIONAL SYSTEMS – MAY BE MORE DIFFICULT TO ASSESS

- Symptoms of imbalance: anxious, bored, scared, mad, sad, depressed, scattered, restless, irritable, agitated, hyped
- Symptoms of balance: confident, excited, humorous, excited, interested, calm, relaxed, focused, easygoing, patient.

Adapted from Potatoes Not Prozac, by Kathleen DesMaisons, PhD.

DAY	Breakfast	Lunch	Snack	Dinner	Snack	Prep
Day 1						
Day 2						
Day 3						
Day 4						
Day 5						
Day 6						

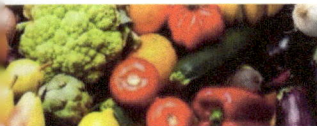

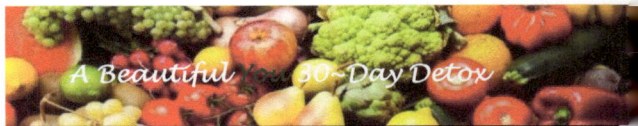

Day 7					
Day 8					
Day 9					
Day 10					
Day 11					
Day 12					
Day 13					
Day 14					
Day 15					

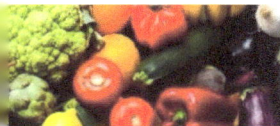

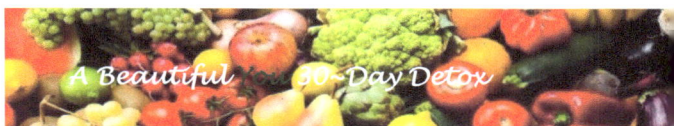

Day 16					
Day 17					
Day 18					
Day 19					
Day 20					
Day 21					
Day 22					
Day 23					
Day 24					
Day 25					

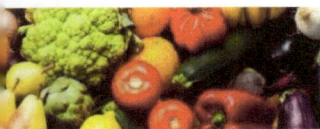

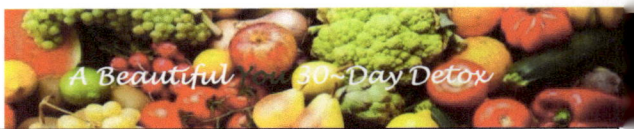

Day 26					
Day 27					
Day 28					
Day 29					
Day 30					

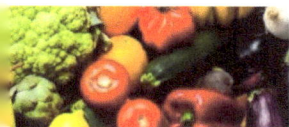

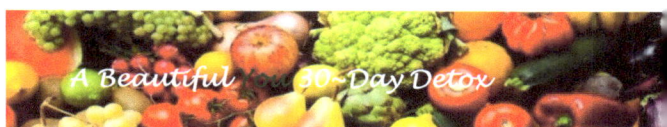

EATING OUT MADE EASY

You may be the type of person that loathes cooking. Or you may just eat out a lot and you don't have the right tools to order in the way that leaves you feeling satiated, existing in balance, losing weight and thriving successfully. Even if you're not succeeding right at that moment, you can learn how! Keep in mind that the same rules apply to eating out as they do when you're eating at home- always combine a good carb with the proper and healthy protein and healthy fat. It can be a little daunting to navigate menus, parties or those days where you're stuck out on the road without a healthy snack. With little mindfulness, preparation and forward thinking it's possible to succeed.

Listed below are a few tips and ideas to help keep you on track while on the Detox Program and for your lifestyle change.

Eating Easily At Home

1. Steaming, sautéing, baking and roasting are quick, easy and basic ways to cook food.
2. Keep it simple! Don't allow what you don't know what to make, make you feel dumbfounded. Just keep it simple by starting out with a real stainless steel pan. I don't advocate using non – stick because some of the non – stick material can over time begin to come up from the pan and be ingested with your food, which can lead to cancer. Add 1 tbsp. EVOO or EVCO and allow it to sit in the pan for a minute on high heat and warm or in the case of the coconut oil, melt. Use your imagination with this by getting creative. Add a few of your favorite veggies and cook them for 2 minutes. Add some garlic and ginger to the pan and cook for another minute or so. Next, add your protein and once it's in the pan, add a pinch of grey sea salt and pepper to taste. Protein takes about 6 – 8 minutes to cook. Try not to overcook but follow the proper temperature guidelines especially for animal protein. Bon Appetit!
3. Consume foods that are easy on your digestion. Simple ingredients mean more energy, less bloat and more nourishment.

Cooking For People Who Do Not Like To Cook!

1. Cook enough so that there will be leftovers. Also, consider freezing portions for an easy grab and to reheat for later.

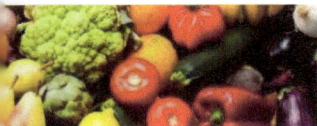

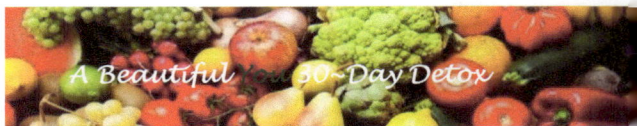

2. It doesn't have to be hard to make time to cook. Begin by trying a few of the delicious recipes in this book and modify them to your liking.

3. Easy meals like protein, veggies and a healthy fat is the key for boosting your metabolism during and after your detox program.

Going To A Deli

When going to a deli, keep in mind that breads are high on the glycemic index. Therefore, choose a broth – base soup with a simple salad and a protein. Your body needs fuel when you begin to crave sweets. Though I don't advocate eating deli meats because of the high amounts of nitrates and sodium, eat sparingly as a condiment on the top of your salad with a little olive oil, vinegar or lemon juice and a pinch of grey sea salt and pepper. Try eating a wrap made of veggies like lettuce, tomato, lean turkey or chicken, avocado spread, or a good salad made with beans or avocado for your Post – Tox days at the deli. Keep in mind that simpler foods produces optimal digestion. Trust me, your belly will thank you!

Your Basic Restaurant Ideas

1. When ordering, get a combination of veggies and proteins
2. Enjoy your meals with simplicity by ordering veggies. Simply ask for them steamed, roasted or sautéed in garlic and olive oil
3. Get the dairy free soup and salad
4. If you're craving carbs, enjoy a sweet potato, some brown rice or red potatoes. Just stay away from the glutens like breads and pastas and foods that are high on the glycemic index. **(See foods low on the glycemic index section).**

Eating Out For Breakfast

For your Post – Tox breakfast, enjoy scramble eggs, egg white omelet with spinach, tomato, garlic, green onion and about 1/3 piece of zucchini or a soft boiled egg. BUT NO CHEESE! NO GOOD FOR DIGESTION!

Oatmeal is a good option, but keep away from the instant oatmeal as it contains sugar. Top with dry fruit and sweeten with agave nectar, raw honey or 100% maple syrup.

If you're a diabetic, try and stay away from coffee and steer towards the herbal teas. But if not, coffee should only be done in moderation and it also should be organic. But if you can also steer clear from it, all the better. Use your better judgment if you decide to drink coffee

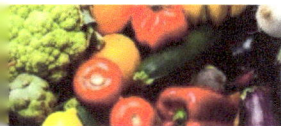

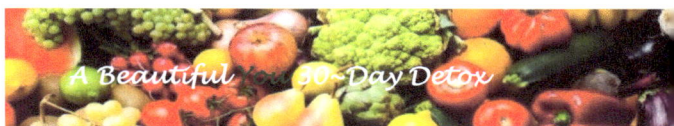

and try keeping it to only 1 cup per day. Use drip coffee and sweeten it with stevia, or another natural sweetener and use almond milk if available at the restaurant.

Fruit Bowls are a great way to get large quantities of fruit along – side a bowl of oatmeal or an omelet.

Unhealthy Foods To Stay Away From

- Processed meats, including breakfast meats. It's not good at all for your body and skin.
- White bread and potatoes because they raise your glycemic index.
- Creamy sauces and dishes because they are loaded with un-healthy fats.
- French toast, pancakes, waffles and pastries. They are loaded with sugars, but if you really want it, order it and split it with your friends or family members and make it a treat day.

Lunch & Dinner At Restaurants

Make sure to choose the salmon, chicken, fish, lean meat or all veggies. Ask for extra veggies instead of the high glycemic carbs. Imagine your plate being ½ veggies, ¼ protein, and ¼ healthy carbs, or you may choose not to have the carbs at all and if you choose a fat, make sure that it's a healthy one. Don't go for the extra sauces as this can un-do all of your hard work and will only cause you to gain that unwanted weight back. Yeah, I know, they are so darn good, but some of them are high in unhealthy fats and sugars that does a body bad.

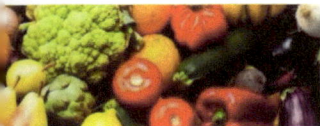

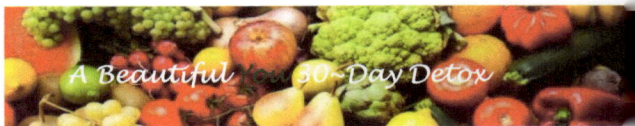

DRINK YOURSELF THIN WITH PROBIOTICS

Diets rich in probiotics add healthy bacteria to your body. The added bacteria to your gut really improves your body's ability to absorb nutrition, boost your immunity, reduce levels of toxicity in your body and also supports a healthy weight loss. Foods fermented are highly beneficial for detoxing.

Making cultured drinks can be very hard work, feel impossible or even scary, but don't fear it. Make it fun and drink yourself thin! Have confidence in yourself, you can do it. Besides, the bacteria not only allows you to drink yourself thin, but it also hydrates you.

Easy Steps for Making Kefir Water

Coconut Water Kefir

- 4 cup glass jar with wide mouth and good screw top or swing away lid
- ¼ cup water kefir grains *you can get them from http://www.culturesforhealth.com/water-kefir-grains.html
- 2 – 4 cups fresh coconut water
  1. Fill the jar with water and coconut water and add water kefir grains. Stir with a non-metal spatula as metal may destroy the grains.
  2. Seal the jar airtight and let stand 24 – 48 hours. The long it sits the more beneficial bacteria you've cultured.
  3. Strain through a coffee filter and fill bottles with coconut water and seal the bottles airtight. Do this all the time for a new batch.

How to make your own natural weight loss detox water

Get rid of toxicity, add nutrients and drink away the weight!

You can add vital nutrients & minerals to your water while flushing away the toxins from your body by following the combinations below:

- ~ ½ gallon water
- ~ 1 grapefruit
- ~ 1 tangerine
- ~ 1 large cucumber, sliced
- ~ 10 – 20 peppermint leaves

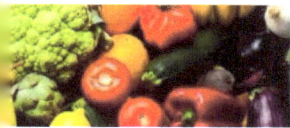

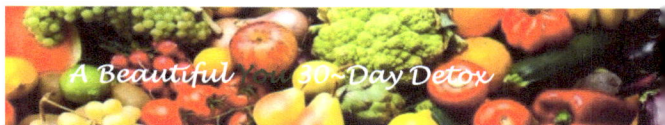

~   As much ice as you want

Method:

Rinse all fruit, cucumber and peppermint leaves. Slice cucumber and fruit. Combine all ingredients in a half gallon jug or pitcher. The longer it sits, the better the benefits.

Here's another easy beneficial drink. Get a large pitcher or other BPH free container and fill it with filtered water. Then add:

~   Fresh fruits, sliced so thin that you could see through it
~   Mint
~   Stevia or raw honey for sweetness

Put your detox water in the fridge for at least 4 – 6 hours and serve over ice.

a.   Green Tea, Mint with Lime – this is a great aid in fat burning and assist with digestion, alleviating headaches, and congestion. Also a great way to freshen your breath.
b.   Strawberry – Kiwi – enhances cardio vascular health, immune protection, regulates blood sugar, helps with digestion.
c.   Cucumber, Lime & Lemon – acts as a diuretic, reduces bloating, controls the appetite, hydrates you, and helps in digestion.
d.   Lemon, Lime & Orange – helps with proper digestion, has vitamin C, supports immune system, relieves heartburn, this one is best served at room temperature.

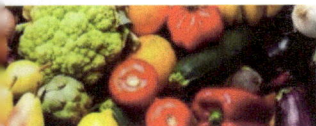

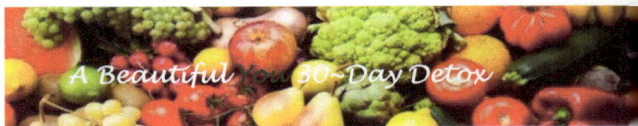

STAGING THE KITCHEN

b.k.a

Prepping for the Detox

One of the biggest obstacles that gets in the way of our achieving our goals is the lack of proper planning and preparation for the journey ahead. This is to be a fun, easy and successful Detox. Proper kitchen staging will be a huge asset in achieving this goal and will also set you on the right path...ditching that diet mentality forever!

Please follow these very easy guidelines to maximize your prep time and ensure that you feel organized and confident in your kitchen. These guidelines are superb for Pre – Tox, during Detox and after your Post – Tox.

Step 1: Plan Your Meals For The WEEK!

Go through the recipe section of this book and choose your meals for the week ahead. Don't mindlessly do this, take your time and do this. Look over the recipes and ask yourself, what looks delicious? What are your cravings? Try writing out your meals on your calendar so that you won't be lost for the week. Keep your schedule in mind when doing this. Do you work late? Do you have meetings during the week? If so, select a dinner that you can heat up in a crock-pot, eat a raw meal, or double-up a recipe. You can also plan ahead by making meals for the week on your day off, I find that this helps me keep to my busy schedule. When you do this, if you have a vacuum sealer, store leftovers in a vacuum sealed pouch and save for later in the week. Don't be dogmatic about it though, because just because you've decided to do a detox doesn't mean that things will start moving at a slower pace. Take the time to really plan your detox out so that you can reach your goals. Begin by planning your meals as this removes the obstacles and last minute questions, "what am I gonna eat" and "how do I get it on the table quick and in a hurry". Remember, this is supposed to be fun and enjoyable and the time that you spend prepping will save you at least twice as much time later on in the week. So don't stress because you want to support your goals, not sabotage them. Plan your week out!

Step 2: Create Your List Only For The Week!

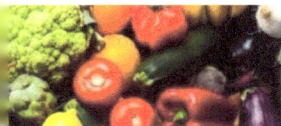

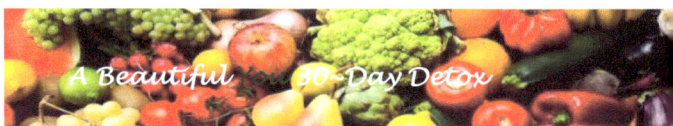

Once you've decided your menu for the week, take into consideration your schedule and the foods you'd prefer, take a look at the ingredients needed and create your shopping list for the week. Vegetables are perishable and they will spoil quickly. When you go to the store, shop only from your list and as the week goes by, this will help you to find and track the foods that are easiest for you to prepare and also keep you feeling satiated, well-nourished and fueled for the day. You'll also notice that shopping from your list only lowers your grocery bill and decreases food waste. Now you know that you'll use the fresh fruits and veggies that you bought by the week's end, because it's on your menu for the week. That's the end of throwing away healthy foods that you bought with the good intentions of eating healthy but never got around to it. Once more, the more you prepare during your Detox and Post – Tox, the easier eating clean foods will be for you. When you plan, prep and prepare, eating clean becomes a whole lot easier and lots more fun. So, choose your menu! Create a shopping list. Now you have a plan!

Step 3: Making Your Dips & Dressings For The Week!

Dips and dressings are a great way to start your weekly kitchen prep after you've done the grocery shopping. Prepare according to the recipe section of this book and then store in the fridge in BPA free containers or glass mason jars. This small accomplishment will put you further down the path of preparation. You'll feel the calm and control begin to set in!

Step 4: Do Your Prepping: Chopping & Peeling For The Week!

Take some time to peel, chop and organize your produce for the week. Choose one day of the week to do this, for me, Sunday is the best day of the week, but you choose which day works for you. Use the recipe section to prepare for the menu that you've selected for the week ahead. This may seem like a daunting task, but it's all worth it. Once you settle in and this becomes routine for you, this step will really feel less like a chore, especially if you're partnering with someone and more like a reward to yourself as the week unfolds. Make it fun, try involving the whole family and make a date of it. Or you can do some me time on a certain week night, whatever works best for you. I know that it seems logical to begin on a Monday, but you can begin your Detox Program any day of the week. Any day of the week is a great day to get into you AND a great day to begin your Detox Program! Now you're ready to begin on your road to success!

Page | 122

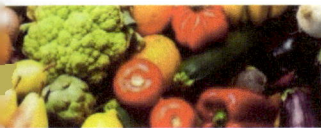

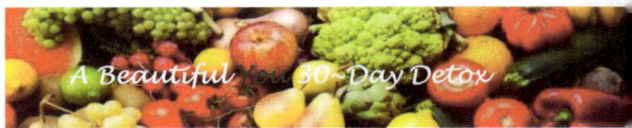

Step 5: Pre – Cook

Set aside some time to pre – cook your proteins for the week and store them in the fridge or freezer. For the Post – Tox, grill, bake or broil your proteins slice side up and store the right portion amount for easy access. If you're vegetarian or vegan, make sure you always have plant-based proteins available. Make your choice to eat healthy as fast, easy and fun as you can!

Step 6: Cook Once, Eat Twice or More!

OK, let's get real here…who has the time to be in the kitchen every-day? I know I don't, so make double, triple or quadruple the recipe for easy leftovers and freezer storage. The plan for the meals in this book is only for suggestions or a model to follow, and remember, no one ever said that dinner had to be different every night of the week. I like leftovers because it gives the seasonings time to marry even better. So if you find a recipe that you especially like and keeps you full, happy and really look forward to sitting down and eating again, go for it! If your day looks to be hectic and busy, then plan for leftovers from last night's dinner or lunch. Just get that portion out of the fridge or freezer and warm it in a small sauce pan with hot water if frozen in a pouch, if in a container, warm in a crock pot. This is great for when you have an unscheduled event to pop up in the week. If you find yourself not able to prepare a meal for that day, then at least you have the satisfaction of knowing that you have a delicious and healthy back-up plan in the fridge or freezer.

Make this Detox Program easy for you by putting some effort in your prep. Following these guidelines is your Detox safety net for those times that may, and most likely will, come up in the week that you simply didn't plan for. You'll feel a great sense of success when life's little mis-haps don't throw off your Detox or game!

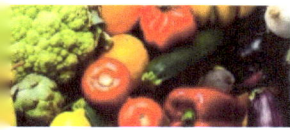

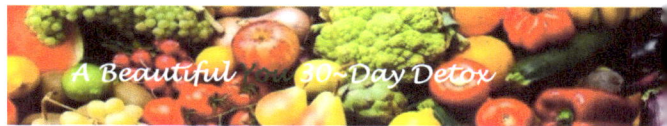

ABOUT THE AUTHOR

How My Journey Began

My journey began at the age of 19...let me go back a few years earlier. I met my husband at 17 years old. Is was so very young and naïve about life. If foolishly thought that I needed a man to take care of me and my son, Corey, and I, don't get me wrong because my husband is the love of my life, didn't know nor did he know what a healthy diet was and we ate anything that was deemed by society as "healthy". In my mind, I thought that I was doing pretty good...I only weighed 98 pounds soaking wet, as they would say.

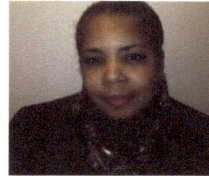

As the years passed, I got pregnant with my second child and in the beginning of the pregnancy, the weight started to creep up on my small frame. I thought that I was eating a healthy diet with my brown foods, right along with my greasy foods. My salty and sweet cravings were through the roof! My idea of a healthy breakfast, being from the south, consisted of grits, eggs, bacon and toast with a huge glass of whatever juice we had in the fridge. "What?" I would say..."I'm eating for two!" was my excuse. With that pregnancy, the weight didn't creep on, it flew on as I continue to ravage my poor little frame with extra weight.

Two years later, my third pregnancy came along and I was bed ridden as I was threatening to miscarry with this pregnancy. Guess what? You guessed it, more weight! After having my beautiful baby girl, Yay, finally a girl, I decided to breast feed her and ate like a garbage disposal! Literally! What was I eating?? Every fried piece of food, every salty thing and all the sweets that I could get my hands on. Never for one moment did I consider the affect that it would have on my baby's health and the quality of milk that I'd produce. The quality was so poor that it did effect the health of my daughter, causing her to go into the hospital. I asked the doctor if this happen because of my diet and his answer, of course, was no. Whew, I thought to myself. I didn't do this to my precious baby girl! Really! Do I seriously believe that? NO!

Four years later, yep you guessed it...I was pregnant again! This time though, I'd do things a little different. Not too healthy for the baby, but different. I went on a twelve hundred calorie a day diet for a while, that is, until my doctor tore into me. After the birth of my last son, I ate poorly so my milk was scarce, leaving me no choice but to bottle feed him

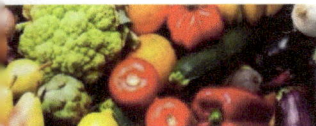

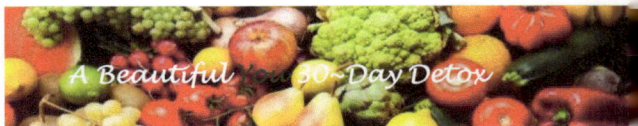

so that he could be sustained. By this time, my weight was 187 pounds. WOW! How I wish that was the case now!

Anyway, fast forward to my 40's, my weight skyrocketed to a whopping 215 pounds. This was the result of my yo-yo dieting. But wait, that wasn't my heaviest! I remember feeling like I did something good by dieting a week before going to the doctor's office only to find out that I'd gained weight! At my heaviest in my 40's, I was 278 pounds. I felt heart broken and deflated. How could I let this happen to me? I'd get comments like: "You're so beautiful, if only you'd lose that fat!" I'd ask my husband, "Honey, how do I look?" and without giving me a glance, he'd say "You look Ok." For a while, I accepted that. But one day I insisted on his taking a look at me and giving me his honest opinion. What he said spoke volumes when he said: "You always look good to me." Or "It doesn't matter, you're old." And he'd chuckle it off. Thing is, I'm not old now and when he was saying it, I wasn't old then. I love him for not wanting to hurt my feelings, but I think that if he'd been honest but tactful, it would have made the world of difference.

Let's fast forward to now-a-days... It gets worse! My weight exploded when I reached a shocking 349 pounds! I was at a loss and didn't know what to do with my diet and weight. I hid the fact that I weighed so much from my husband. I was on tons of medications for my high blood pressure, cholesterol and was border line diabetic. I was stumped because the doctors kept telling me to go on a bland food diet. What! A bland diet! That's what got me in hot water with my weight in the past. I'd go on a bland diet only to gain the weight back and then some.

OK, I was living with my weight. When I began going to my religious weekly meetings, I met this lady there and I must say that she was a very interesting person to say the least. What she had to tell me BLEW my mind because she had a wealth of information and was very knowledgeable when it came to healthy eating. "OK, not one doctor has ever told me the things that she was telling me" was my thought. Thing was, she never tried to ogle me or force any of her dietary beliefs on me. I found myself having to pick her brain! I follower her around like a little lost puppy, eager for more healthy information. Once she saw that I was serious, totally interested and eager to learn more, the flood gates opened! What I'd learned from her lead me to take a course in integrative nutrition.

Being serious about my diet and wanting to share with others what I'd learned, I signed up for a course at Institute for Integrative Nutrition in 2012 and became a Certified Holistic Health Coach. But I still struggled with my weight and couldn't figure out which eating

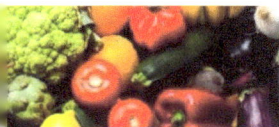

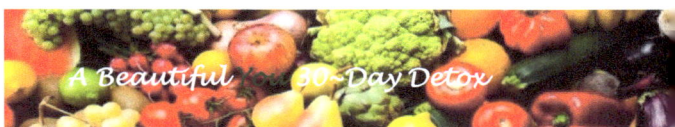

plan was right for me. Meanwhile, I'm dealing with breakouts all over my body, so I went to the doctor only to find out that I'm dealing with a severe case of Candida Overgrowth. Where did that come from, I wondered and where do I go from there. Well, I did my research and took it from there! This lead to my 30 ~ Day Detox Program. I truly thought that eating raw was going to kill me until I started searching the internet for recipes……and find them I did. Being from New Orleans, you know that I had to tweak them to give them that Creole flare, making them my own and guess what? They taste fantastic! I also found out through being rushed to the hospital several times that I have a severe case of Crohn's disease. It's so severe that I cannot digest meat any more. No steak, chicken or fowl of any kind, lamb, pork or goat! NO MEAT PERIOD! Doctors say that give it some time and I may not be able to eat fish anymore. Mom told me that I was that way as a baby, but I grew out of it, but guess what….it's back with a vengeance!

Being on my own Detox Program has allotted me the opportunity to lose weight and feel healthier! My arthritis is a thing of the past, my blood pressure has dropped significantly, and I'm no longer taking cholesterol medication and am no longer border line diabetic! Although most of the foods on the program are raw, there are a few that are not! That's ok, though, you're looking for that alkalinity. I promise you that with all of the delicious recipes, you won't get bored. Please enjoy your journey, have fun doing your Detox and watch as the weight melts off!

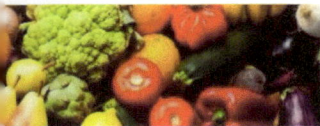

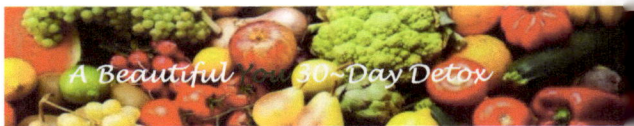

KUDOS AND THANK YOUS

I'd like to thank my husband, Tom, whose support is almost never ending. Linda Simmons, because had it not been for her, none of this would've taken place. Joellen Rousse, whose friendship and support is phenomenal and never ending. Mrs. Vanessa Ross, thank you Vanna for helping me get this valuable information out and was there for me even from your bed and most of all, thank you Rachel Feldman for helping me write this book.

DEDICATION

This book is dedicated to my husband, Tom Riley Sr., without whose support, none of this would have taken shape. You were my first guinea pig. If it was bad, you'd let me know. To my daughter, Tandra Hughes, whose loving words pushed me forward when I was stressed. My son, Chris, who provided me with ways of getting around to seminars and gave me his valuable input. Tommy Riley Jr., for running me to the store at all hours of the night or day even at inconvenient times to buy what I needed to test my recipes. My brother, Karl Jones, for running me around when Tommy Jr. wasn't around to do so. Tia Geanette, who was also one of my guinea pigs and was pleasantly surprised. Corey Riley just for being himself. Linda Simmons, she kept me on my toes and made sure things were delicious. Without you guys, none of this could have happened. I thank and love all of you guys for all of your help!

www.ingramcontent.com/pod-product-compliance
Lightning Source LLC
Chambersburg PA
CBHW040512290326
R18043100001B/R180431PG41927CBX00003B/3